JN013051

Basic English

医療従事者のための
ベーシックイングリッシュ

小澤 淑子 [編] ／ Michael E. Lawson [英語監修]

for
Health Care
Workers

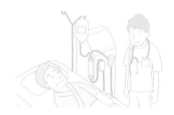

Ohmsha

編者・執筆者等一覧

| 編　者 | 小澤　　淑子（鈴鹿医療科学大学） |
| 英語監修 | Michael E. Lawson（鈴鹿工業高等専門学校） |

執　筆　者　片岡　由美子（愛知県立大学）
　　　　　　小澤　　淑子（鈴鹿医療科学大学）
　　　　　　高木　　久代（鈴鹿医療科学大学）
　　　　　　服部　しのぶ（藤田医科大学）
　　　　　　平井　　聡子（鈴鹿医療科学大学）

医学監修　　亀山　洋一郎（愛知学院大学、藤田医科大学）
　　　　　　藤原　奈佳子（人間環境大学）

医療従事者のためのベーシックイングリッシュ（第1版第1刷）正誤表

頁	該当箇所／行	誤	正
15	MT内	（追加）	cartilage 軟骨
24	3	breakdown	break down
43	RC6	visiting	visiting
47	MT内	cartilage 軟骨	（削除）
49	24〜26	厚い軟骨で守られた喉頭と、C字型の連続した⑤＿＿を持つ気管は共に決して塞がらない。これらは呼吸器官の壁から分泌される⑥＿＿で覆われておりこの膜は呼吸の際、……	厚い⑤＿＿で守られた喉頭と、C字型の連続した⑤＿＿を持つ気管は共に決して塞がらない。これらは呼吸器官の壁の膜から分泌される⑥＿＿で覆われている。この⑥は呼吸の際、……
49	30	粘液	粘膜
57	Figure2	renal tuble	renal tubule
73	MT内	stimuli 刺激	stimulus 刺激 （複数形はstimuli）
74	2	agonistic	antagonistic
91	MT内	弾性繊維	弾性繊維
100	22	pancreases that are	pancreas that is
109	RC2	uterine tube	fallopian tube
109	RC4	antigen	an antigen
118	RC6	are two	are the two
118	16	leukemia	leucocyte
118	16	leukemia	leucocyte
119	1	dose	does
129	23	⑥粘液	⑥粘膜
129	26	4. mucous, respiratory, tissues	4. mucous, air, tissues
139	30	leukemia	leucocyte
140	10	⑤自己免疫系	⑤自然免疫系

※MT：Medical terminology，RC：Reading Comprehension

オーム社／ISBN:978-4-274-22489-8

はじめに

　医療英語というと、診療時や病棟での定型的な会話をイメージすることが多いと思います。しかし、医療に関わる学習者の方からは、もう少し切り口の異なる医療に関係した英会話を学びたいという要望も多く聞きます。また、医療分野で働く様々な専門家について、英語学習を通して知ってもらうことは、医療の専門家にとっては相互理解を深めるために重要であり、一般の人々にとっては馴染みのない専門職について知る貴重な機会ともなります。さらに、英語について様々な思いをもつ学習者が共に学ぶための教材として、解剖生理学の基礎を扱った英文は学習者の知的好奇心に訴え、大きな学習動機となるものと考えます。

　本書の対話文では、家庭や身の回りで交わされる生きた日常会話の中で、健康問題の基本情報を得られるようにしました。これに端を発し、健康に問題をもつ人と医療の専門家との臨場感のある会話へと発展させ、会話から医療の専門家の特徴が学べるように工夫しています。

　解剖生理学の内容はまとまった英文読解の学習に役立つものと思います。解剖生理学をよく理解している方にとっては、内容に関する知識が英語の学習の助けとなります。また、そこで扱われている専門用語はかなり難しいレベルとなっており、英語の得意な人にとっても文脈の中で飽きることなく的確な英語の知識を獲得していただけるでしょう。

　このように、本書は様々な背景をもつ読者の要望に応えられるよう、亀山洋一郎先生、藤原奈佳子先生の医学的な内容監修のもと、執筆者一同、英語として自然な表現を繰り返し追求した一冊です。そのための長い道のりを辛抱強くご支援いただきましたオーム社編集局の方々には心より感謝申し上げます。

2020 年 3 月

編　者

＜本書の特徴＞

Medical Terminology:
　　　　　専門性が高いが日常で頻用されるものを習得できる。

Reading Comprehension:
　　　　　自習やペアワークに活用しやすく、自然に内容の把握ができる。

対話文：　前半、後半で区切った学習ができる。
　　　　　ト書きで前半、後半のそれぞれの状況を理解しやすい。
　　　　　（前半では家族・友人間の日常会話で健康問題を提起）
　　　　　（後半では一般人と医療の専門家の会話で専門的な内容を説明）

Exercise:　正誤問題や内容の要約の空所補充問題で理解した内容の復習に活用できる。

語彙：　　多くの専門用語も文脈で理解でき、難しい語彙も覚えやすい。

Reading Comprehension:
　　　　　グループワークで利用すると自然に内容の理解が確認できる。

本文：　　英語構文も論理性も理解しやすく多様な学習者に適している。

Figure:　解剖の知識で英文理解を深められる。

Exercise:　正誤問題や内容に関する多様な空所補充問題で復習に活用しやすい。

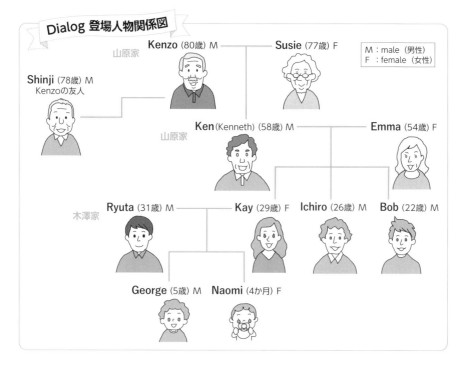

Dialog 登場人物関係図

目次　v

目 次

CONTENTS

はじめに iii

Unit 1
Regions of the Body
【身体の部位】 **1**

Dialog
Receptionists and Health Insurance 1

Anatomy and Physiology
Regions of the Body.. 5

Unit 2
The Skeletal and Muscular System
【筋肉系・骨格系】 **11**

Dialog
Osteoporosis and Occupational Therapists 11

Anatomy and Physiology
The Skeletal and Muscular System 15

<音声データダウンロードサービスについて>
本書籍発刊に伴い、各Unitの英語音声データのダウンロードサービスを開始する予定です。
詳細につきましては、オーム社HP（https://www.ohmsha.co.jp/book/9784274224898/）
にてご確認ください。

Unit 1

Regions of the Body

【身体の部位】

本課の ねらい	Dialog	健康診断や健康保険、受付に関する表現が使える。
	Anatomy and Physiology	身体の部位、身体の方向や位置に関する英語表現を理解する。

Dialog ── Receptionists and Health Insurance

Medical Terminology

abdominal ultrasound	腹部超音波検査	health insurance card	健康保険証 (カード)
application form	申込用紙		
EGD (esophagogastroduodenoscopy)		medical checkup	健康診断
	上部消化管内視鏡検査	sample	検体、検査試料
		urine	尿
fecal occult blood test	便潜血検査	X-ray	レントゲン (検査)
gastroscopy	胃カメラ、胃内視鏡検査		

Reading Comprehension

Based on the dialog below, please answer the following questions.

1. Why wasn't Emma able to eat or drink anything?
2. Why did Emma choose the stomach X-ray instead of the gastroscopy?
3. What will Emma bring to the hospital?
4. Where will Emma take the urine sample?
5. What kind of health insurance does Emma have?
6. Where is the medical checkup center?
7. What time is Emma's appointment for her medical checkup?
8. Will Emma have an EGD instead of an X-ray?

Emma (54 years old) is preparing for her yearly medical checkup and talking with her son Bob (22 years old). Emma (54歳) は、息子のBob (22歳) と話しながら毎年の健康診断を受けるための準備をしている。

Bob： Why didn't you eat anything this morning?

Emma： I'll have a medical checkup today.

Bob： Oh, I remember you were wondering what type of checkup you would have.

Emma： Yes. I added a stomach X-ray test and an abdominal ultrasound to the usual checkup.

Bob： Didn't you choose the gastroscopy instead of the stomach X-ray?

Emma： The gastroscopy seems to be so popular that they couldn't schedule me for two months.

Bob： Really? Can you wait for two months?

Emma： I want to finish the checkup be-fore traveling with Ken.

Bob： Stop, Mom! You can't drink anything, can you?

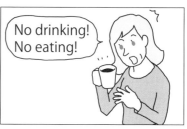

Emma： Woops. I nearly drank coffee.

Bob： You'd better leave now, other-wise you might end up eating or drinking something.

Emma： Yes, it's almost time to go. I must bring my samples for the fecal occult blood test I prepared, and the application form.

Bob： Have you taken the urine sample?

Emma： No. I'll take that in the hospital. Oh, I must bring the health insurance card, too.

Bob： Will the medical checkup be covered by health insurance?

Emma： No, but I think they need it for identification.

Bob： I see. By the way, what kind of health insurance do you have? I had the opportunity to learn about the Japanese health insurance system and am interested in your case.

Emma： I am covered by Ken's company's insurance.

Bob： That means you are covered as a family member of your husband's employee health insurance.

Emma： That's right. I need to go now.

Bob： OK. Good luck!

Emma is talking to a hospital receptionist (Recp). Emmaは病院の受付係と話している。

Recp： Good morning. How can I help you?

Emma： Hi, I'm going to have a complete medical checkup.

Recp： Do you have an appointment?

Emma： Yes. Here's the copy of the application form.

Recp： OK. Then will you go to the fifth floor? The medical checkup center is there.

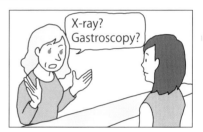

Emma： I see. Where is the elevator?

Recp： Can you see an escalator over there? An elevator is behind the escalator.

Emma： Thank you.

At the reception desk on the fifth floor. 5階の受付で

Recp： Hello. Are you going to have a medical checkup?

Emma： Yes. I have an appointment for 9 o'clock today.

Recp： May I ask your name please?

Emma： I'm Emma Yamahara. Here's my health insurance card.

Recp： Thank you. Have you eaten or consumed any liquid this morning?

Emma： No. I haven't had anything since 11 o'clock last night.

Recp： OK. You are going to have a stomach X-ray and an abdominal ultrasound in addition to the regular course, right?

Emma：It is impossible to take the gastroscopy, isn't it?

Recp：Do you prefer the gastroscopy to the X-ray?

Emma：Yes. I had to take the gastroscopy after having the stomach X-ray last year.

Recp：After receiving the X-ray result, it is recommended that some take the EGD.

Emma：Does EGD mean gastroscopy?

Recp：Yes. EGD stands for esophagogastroduodenoscopy.

Emma：I see. The EGD covers the esophagus and duodenum as well as the stomach, doesn't it? I couldn't make an appointment for the EGD today. That's why I chose the stomach X-ray.

Recp：There was a cancellation today so let me check...Oh, you can have the EGD this morning.

Emma：That's lucky. I've really wanted to have that.

Recp：OK. Would you come this way?

Exercise 1.　Indicate True or False based on the dialog.

会話文の内容に合っていれば T、合っていなければ F と記入しなさい。

( ) 1.　Emma could not wait for two months to have the gastroscopy.

( ) 2.　Emma drank coffee this morning.

( ) 3.　Emma's medical checkup will be covered by health insurance.

( ) 4.　Emma had not had any food or drink for about 10 hours when she arrived at the hospital.

( ) 5.　The EGD is recommended for every person after taking the stomach X-ray.

Exercise 2.　Fill in the blanks of the receptionist's memo with words from the word list.

次の受付係のメモの空所に適する語を下の語群より選び、記入しなさい。

For this year, Ms. Yamahara actually had hoped to book (1.   ) instead of a stomach X-ray to avoid the possibility of having to (2.   ) both the X-ray and the EGD like last year. However, she couldn't make (3.   ) to suit her convenience and she unwillingly chose (4.   ). Luckily for her, there was (5.   ) of the EGD and she was happy to (6.   ) her test items from an X-ray to the EGD.

Word list: an appointment, a cancellation, change, an EGD, take, an X-ray

Anatomy and Physiology   Regions of the Body

Medical Terminology

abdomen	腹部	nervous	神経の
anatomy	解剖学	organ	器官
anterior	前方(の)	palmar	手掌(の)、掌側(の)
caudal	尾側(の)	pelvis	骨盤
cell	細胞	perineum	会陰
circulatory	循環器の	plantar	足底(の)
cranial	頭側	posterior	後方(の)
digestive	消化器の	posture	姿勢
dorsal	背側(の)	reproductive	生殖器の
dorsum	背	respiratory	呼吸器の
endocrine	内分泌の	sensory	感覚の
immune	免疫の	skeletal	骨格の
inferior	下方(の)、下位(の)	superior	上方(の)、上位(の)
lateral	外側(の)	system	系、器官系
longitudinally	縦に	thorax	胸部
lower limb	下肢	tissue	組織
medial	内側(の)	upper limb	上肢
median plane	正中面	urinary	泌尿器の
muscular	筋肉の	ventral	腹側(の)

Reading Comprehension

Based on the text below, please answer the following questions.

1. In terms of anatomy, what is the smallest unit of the body?
2. What are the eleven organ systems dealt with in this text?
3. Besides body-part names, what do health care professionals need to know in order to study the organ systems?
4. How can the body be divided by regions?
5. Which structures of the body does "ventral" refer to?
6. Which structures of the body does "caudal" refer to?
7. What plane can divide the body into right and left halves?
8. How can you describe the position of "palm" in reference to the hand in anatomy?

      Anatomy is the study of the structure of the body. In human anatomy, the smallest unit is the cell. Although the components of each cell are almost identical, their shapes and sizes vary. The body's tissues, composed of cells of similar type, constitute organs which comprise internal systems. Systems can be categorized as skeletal, muscular, digestive, circulatory (including blood), respiratory, nervous, urinary, sensory (including skin), reproductive, endocrine, and the immune system. This textbook addresses these systems.

      When studying these systems, medical professionals often refer to sections of the body using various technical terms to describe a specific body part. To understand anatomy, we need to know not only the technical terms of the body parts, but also the terms of position and direction.

      Dividing the body into regions is one way to describe body parts. The regions can consist of the head and neck, the upper limbs, the back, the chest or thorax, the abdomen, the perineum, the pelvis, and the lower limbs. Another way to describe the body is by using the concept of positions or directions. Anterior (ventral) means structures nearer to the front of the body, while posterior (dorsal) refers to structures nearer to the back of the body. Superior (cranial) refers to the structures nearer to the head, and inferior (caudal) means nearer to the feet.

Moreover, imaginary planes are drawn through the body at different parts in order to provide separation into various sections. For example, the median plane passes longitudinally, dividing the body into right and left halves. Medial refers to nearer to the median plane of the body, and conversely, lateral indicates farther away from the median plane.

In anatomy, the body is described in a standing posture with the arms hanging by the sides and the eyes looking forward horizontally with the palms of the hands directed forward. So, the palmar surface of the hand (palm) is anterior to the dorsal surface (back) of the hand. The plantar surface (lower) is inferior to the dorsum (upper) of the foot.

Figure 1. 身体の部位と断面に関して、空所に適切な英語、あるいは日本語を記入しなさい。

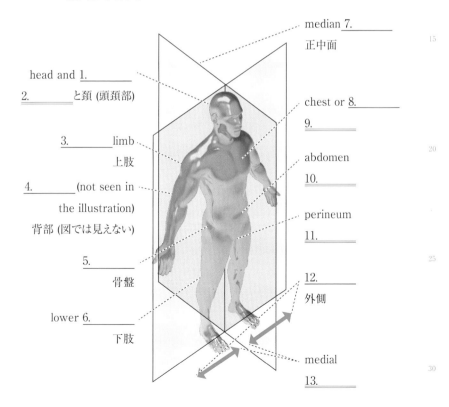

median 7.＿＿＿＿＿
正中面

head and 1.＿＿＿＿＿
2.＿＿＿＿＿と頚 (頭頚部)

chest or 8.＿＿＿＿＿
9.＿＿＿＿＿

3.＿＿＿＿＿limb
上肢

abdomen
10.＿＿＿＿＿

4.＿＿＿＿＿(not seen in
the illustration)
背部 (図では見えない)

perineum
11.＿＿＿＿＿

5.＿＿＿＿＿
骨盤

12.＿＿＿＿＿
外側

lower 6.＿＿＿＿＿
下肢

medial
13.＿＿＿＿＿

Figure 2.　解剖学で方向や位置関係に関して、空所に適切な英語、あるいは日本語を記入しなさい。

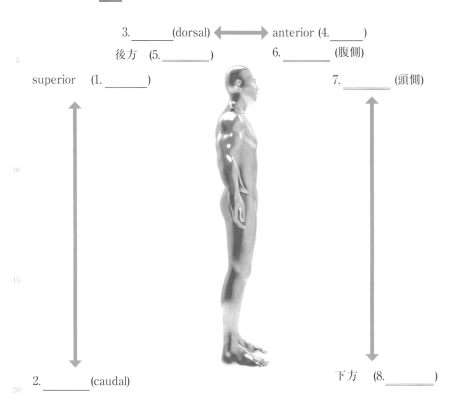

3.＿＿＿＿(dorsal) ⟷ anterior (4.＿＿＿＿)

後方　(5.＿＿＿＿)　　　6.＿＿＿＿(腹側)

superior　(1.＿＿＿＿)　　　　　　　7.＿＿＿＿(頭側)

2.＿＿＿＿(caudal)

下方　(8.＿＿＿＿)

Exercise 1.　本文の要約となるように下の語群より適語を選び、空所を補充しなさい。

　人体の最小単位は①＿＿＿＿であり、似たような①が集まって②＿＿＿＿を形成し、さまざまな②が集まって③＿＿＿＿を構成している。さらにいくつかの③が集まって例えば循環器系、呼吸器系といった④＿＿＿＿を形成し、機能している。

　人体を表す表現として、人体の部位に分ける方法があるが、その場合は頭部、頸部、上肢、背部、胸部、腹部、会陰、骨盤、⑤＿＿＿＿などに分けられる。

　身体の位置を示すために、医療分野では専門的な表現を用いる。例えば、体の

1

前面に近いところを指す場合⑥「＿＿＿＿＿」と言い、背部に近いところを指す場合
は⑦「＿＿＿＿＿」と言い、頭部に近いところを⑧「＿＿＿＿＿」、足部に近い方を⑨
「＿＿＿＿＿」と言う。また、身体を左右に分ける面を⑩「＿＿＿＿＿」と呼び、⑩に近
いところを「内側」、⑩から遠いところを⑪「＿＿＿＿＿」と言う。解剖学においては、
人体を腕は体側で手掌を前方へ向けて直立しているとし、手掌は手の甲より⑥で、
足底は足背より⑫「＿＿＿＿＿」ということになる。

> 語群：器官、器官系、下肢、正中面、組織、細胞、前方、後方、下方、頭側、外側、
> 尾側

Exercise 2. 人体の系統に関する英語を完成させ、日本語を記入しなさい。

1. the skeletal system　　　　　骨格系
2. the d＿＿＿＿＿ system　　　　＿＿＿＿＿系
3. the r＿＿＿＿＿ system　　　　＿＿＿＿＿系
4. the n＿＿＿＿＿ system　　　　＿＿＿＿＿系
5. the c＿＿＿＿＿ system　　　　＿＿＿＿＿系
6. the u＿＿＿＿＿ system　　　　＿＿＿＿＿系
7. the s＿＿＿＿＿ system　　　　＿＿＿＿＿系
8. the rep＿＿＿＿＿ system　　　＿＿＿＿＿系
9. the e＿＿＿＿＿ system　　　　＿＿＿＿＿系
10. the i＿＿＿＿＿ system　　　　＿＿＿＿＿系
11. the m＿＿＿＿＿ system　　　　＿＿＿＿＿系

Unit 2 The Skeletal and Muscular System
【筋肉系・骨格系】

2

本課の ねらい	Dialog	骨粗鬆症と作業療法士に関する表現が使える。
	Anatomy and Physiology	筋肉と骨の種類と役割に関する英語表現を理解する。

Dialog　Osteoporosis and Occupational Therapists

Medical Terminology

absorb	吸収する	orthopedic	整形外科の
calcium	カルシウム	orthopedic surgeon	整形外科医
compression fracture	圧迫骨折	osteoporosis	骨粗鬆症
diarrhea	下痢	prescribe	処方する
medication	薬物療法、投薬	ultraviolet	紫外線
occupational therapist	作業療法士(OT)	vitamin	ビタミン

Reading Comprehension

Based on the dialog below, please answer the following questions.

1. What kind of doctor is an orthopedic surgeon?
2. Who can give Susie advice about what exercise she should do?
3. Will Susie's back be as straight as it was without surgery?
4. How should Susie make her bones stronger?
5. Besides some exercises at home, what did the OT suggest that Susie do in her daily life?
6. What does the OT suggest to Susie about taking calcium?
7. What is the difference between vitamins D and K?
8. Why is sunlight also important for the bones?

Susie (77 years old) reminds her great-grandson George (5 years old) of his posture and is talking about how to be stronger. Susie(77歳)が ひ 孫 の George(5歳)の姿勢の悪さを注意し、どうしたら強くなれるか話し合っている。

5　Susie：　You have poor posture, George. Straighten yourself up.

George：No. I like this way. Great-grandma's back is round like a kitten's!

Susie：　George, I want to straighten my back but I can't. Can't you stretch your back?

10　George：Yes, I can!

Susie：　That's great!

George：Why can't you straighten your back, Great-grandma?

Susie：　I was told by an orthopedic surgeon that the bones of my back have
15　changed.

George：An orthopedic surgeon?

Susie：　A medical doctor who treats the bones and muscles.

George：Oh, I know. Grandpa went there when he broke his bone.

Susie：　That's right. Grandpa broke his leg when he fell down, I must be care-
20　ful not to fall down.

George：If I play at home, my mom tells me to play outside to become bigger and stronger.

Susie：　That's true. It is good to run about and play catch in the park.

George：OK. Let's jump rope, shall we?

25　Susie：　That's difficult for me. I may fall down and break my bones.

George：I often fall down but I never break my bones.

Susie：　You are young, and your bones are strong enough.

George：Dad always tells me milk makes my bones strong. Don't you drink milk?

30　Susie：　 I drink milk every day. I also eat fish and cheese.

George：Isn't milk good enough for you? What can you do?

Susie： I will ask the occupational therapist what I should do next time.

George： Is an occupational therapist a medical doctor too?

Susie： No, but he gives me advice about what exercises I should do.

George： That's good.

Susie is talking to the occupational therapist (OT). Susieは作業療法士(OT)と話している。

Susie： I was told that I had a compression fracture. The doctor recommended surgery but I don't want to have surgery.

OT： Well, your back will not be as straight as it was without surgery. So, let's try not to make the osteoporosis worse.

Susie： What should I do to make my bones stronger?

OT： There are three points: medication, exercise and diet.

Susie： The doctor prescribed calcium, vitamin D and vitamin K. I'm taking them regularly.

OT： How about exercise? You learned how to exercise last time. Do you have any pain while exercising? Do you exercise daily?

Susie： I could not exercise at home. I'm afraid I will get worse again without your help.

OT： If you feel pain again, you should stop exercising but you can do some exercise safely at home. In addition, you can walk to some places in your daily life.

Susie： I see. I try to exercise and walk to my son's house to see my great-grandchildren.

OT： Are you careful about your meals?

Susie： Yes, I try to take as much calcium as possible. I keep drinking milk every day though I have diarrhea when I drink milk.

OT： Do you usually drink cold milk?

Susie： Yes. I thought warming milk may decrease its nutritional value.

OT： If you have diarrhea, hot milk will be better for you.

Susie： Really? That's good since I prefer hot milk to cold milk.

5 OT： Calcium is included in various foods. Please take calcium from a variety of food on this list. Moreover, don't forget to take vitamins D and K. Vitamin D helps our body absorb the calcium and vitamin K develops bone formation.

Susie： I'll look for food with vitamins D and K on the list too.

10 OT： At the same time, sunlight is important for the bones because vitamin D is produced by the sun's ultraviolet light.

Susie： Thank you for your advice. I will get sunlight by walking to such places as the supermarket and my son's house and try to take many kinds of food with calcium and vitamins.

15

Exercise 1. **Indicate True or False based on the dialog.**
会話文の内容に合っていれば T、合っていなければ F と記入しなさい。

( ) 1. George could not straighten his back because of osteoporosis.

20 ( ) 2. Susie agreed to jump rope with her great-grandson.

( ) 3. Susie drinks milk in spite of diarrhea caused by milk.

( ) 4. Susie should not do exercise by herself without the OT's instruction.

( ) 5. Ultraviolet light is useful to make bones strong.

25 **Exercise 2.** **Fill in the blanks of the following OT's report with words on the word list.**
次の OT の記録の空所を語群の語で埋めなさい。

Susie has no (1.　) and wants to improve her (2.　). She takes her (3.　) and

30 tries to have good (4.　), however, her (5.　) about getting worse prevented her from (6.　). After some explanation, she showed her (7.　) to exercise.

Word list: anxiety, exercising, osteoporosis, pain, will, meals, medication

2

Anatomy and Physiology **The Skeletal and Muscular System**

Medical Terminology

bone marrow	骨髄	movable	可動の
cardiac muscle	心筋	peristalsis	蠕動
clavicle	鎖骨	phalange	指骨
compact bone	緻密骨	phosphorus	リン
contract	収縮する	radius	橈骨
contraction	収縮	rib	肋骨
digestive tract	消化管	scapula	肩甲骨 (複数形は scapulae)
femur	大腿骨	shaft	(長骨の)骨幹
flat bone	扁平骨	skeletal muscle	骨格筋
humerus	上腕骨	skull	頭蓋骨
involuntary	不随意の	smooth muscle	平滑筋
joint	関節	spongy bone	海綿骨
layer	層	striated	横紋のある、横紋筋の
ligament	靭帯	tendon	腱
locomotion	運動	ulna	尺骨
long bone	長骨	unstriated	横紋のない、平滑な
mineral salt	無機塩	voluntary	随意の

Reading Comprehension

Based on the text below, please answer the following questions.

1. What are the three types of muscles in the human body?
2. Which muscles are striated?
3. What is skeletal muscle attached to?
4. Where can smooth muscle be seen?
5. How many bones are there in an adult human body?
6. What organ system is bone cartilage and ligaments part of?
7. What do bones produce in the marrow?
8. Based on shape, ribs are classified as what kind of bones?

A muscle is an organ responsible for bodily movement and the muscular system is composed of all the muscles of the body. All bodily movement, whether visible or not, is helped by muscle contractions. There are three types of muscles in the human body: cardiac, smooth, and skeletal. According to the other classification based on the different types of muscle tissue, the skeletal and cardiac muscles are striated and the smooth muscle is unstriated.

Muscle that is attached to bone is categorized as skeletal muscle. Whether you are closing your eyes or bending your knees, you are using skeletal muscle. When skeletal muscle contracts, which is a voluntary movement, bones move accordingly. Skeletal muscle is the most common type of muscle in the body. Smooth muscle can be found in the walls of internal organs such as the stomach and intestines. The repeated wave-like muscle contractions in the digestive tracts create involuntary movements called peristalsis, helping break food into small pieces. Cardiac muscle is present only in the heart and pumps blood through the body in a rhythmic manner. Like smooth muscle, it contracts involuntarily.

The skeletal system consists of bones, cartilage, joints, ligaments and other tissues, and it plays an important role in the human body. There are 206 in the adult human body. Bones serve many functions: Bones a) enable body movements by acting together with muscles and components of the skeletal system such as cartilage, joints and ligaments, b) support body parts, such as the central nervous system and lungs, as a framework, c) produce blood cells in the marrow, and d) work as mineral storage mainly calcium and phosphorus.

Bones can be classified into several types according to shape. One example is long bones. The shaft of a long bone is a tube of compact bone containing bone marrow. Long bones include the humerus, femur, radius, ulna and others. Another example is flat bones. Flat bones consist of spongy bone and compact bone—spongy bone is sandwiched by two thin layers of compact bone. The scapulae, ribs and skull are classified as flat bones.

Figure 1. 筋肉について空所に適切な<u>英語</u>、あるいは<u>日本語</u>を記入しなさい。

muscle name	location	tissues (striated or unstriated)	voluntary or involuntary	other features
1._____ muscle 骨格筋	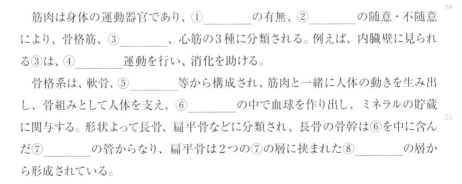	striated 4._____	7._____ 随意筋	most common type of muscle in the body
2._____ muscle 心筋		5._____ 横紋あり	involuntary 8._____	rhythmic contraction
3._____ muscle 平滑筋		6._____ 横紋なし	9._____ 不随意筋	peristalsis 10._____ (repeated wave-like contraction)

Exercise 1. 本文の要約となるように、下の語群から適語を選び空所に記入しなさい。

　筋肉は身体の運動器官であり、①_____の有無、②_____の随意・不随意により、骨格筋、③_____、心筋の3種に分類される。例えば、内臓壁に見られる③は、④_____運動を行い、消化を助ける。

　骨格系は、軟骨、⑤_____等から構成され、筋肉と一緒に人体の動きを生み出し、骨組みとして人体を支え、⑥_____の中で血球を作り出し、ミネラルの貯蔵に関与する。形状よって長骨、扁平骨などに分類され、長骨の骨幹は⑥を中に含んだ⑦_____の管からなり、扁平骨は2つの⑦の層に挟まれた⑧_____の層から形成されている。

　語群：海綿骨、骨髄、横紋、緻密骨、蠕動、収縮、靭帯、平滑筋

Exercise 2.　骨格系のうち、長骨と扁平骨について<u>日本語</u>と<u>英語</u>でまとめましょう。

	構造／structures	骨名の具体例／names of bones
長骨	【外】① _____ 【内】② _____	③ _____ 大腿骨 橈骨（とうこつ） 尺骨
long bone	【Outer】a tube of ④ _____ _____ 【Inner】⑤ _____ _____	humerus ⑥ _____ ⑦ _____ ⑧ _____
扁平骨	【外】⑨ _____ 【内】⑩ _____	⑪ _____ 肋骨 頭蓋骨
flat bone	【Outer】thin layers of ⑫ _____ _____ 【Inner】a layer of ⑬ _____ _____	scapula ⑭ _____ ⑮ _____

Unit 3
The Digestive System
【消化器系】

本課の ねらい	Dialog	便秘、歯周病や歯科衛生士に関する表現が使える。
	Anatomy and Physiology	消化器の臓器と働きに関する英語表現を理解する。

Dialog　Constipation and Dental Hygienists

Medical Terminology

constipate	便秘させる	empty the bowels	通じがある
dental calculus	歯石	enema	浣腸
dental hygienist	歯科衛生士	have a bowel movement	通じがある
dental plaque	デンタルプラーク、歯垢	laxative	下剤
		periodontal disease	歯周病
dental technologist	歯科技工士	scale	(歯石)を取る
denture	入れ歯、義歯		

poop（排便する）、tummy（おなか）は幼児語、belly は abdomen の意味だが口語的

Reading Comprehension

Based on the dialog below, please answer the following questions.

1. Why doesn't Emma feel like eating?
2. What can George do to his grandmother's stomach to help relieve her constipation?
3. What will Emma do before going to see a doctor?
4. How do vegetables help empty our bowels?
5. When is Emma going to see a dentist?
6. What is the role of a dental hygienist?
7. Who makes and fixes dentures?
8. How is the dental calculus of Emma's teeth described?

Emma (54 years old) and George (5 years old) are talking about Emma's constipation and toothache. Emma (54歳) は George(5歳)と便秘や歯痛について話し合っている。

Emma： I don't feel like eating today.

George： Are you sick?

Emma： No. I haven't had a bowel movement for a few days.

George： What is that, Grandma?

Emma： It means poop. I cannot empty my bowels, so my tummy is full. That means I'm constipated.

George： I will warm your tummy with my hands as mom does for me.

Emma： It is really good to warm or massage the belly when we are constipated.

George： You should go to see a doctor.

Emma： Well, if it happens often, I will see a doctor. I think it is not so serious and I can do something before seeing a doctor.

George： What will you do?

Emma： I will drink much water and take a laxative, which is medicine for constipation.

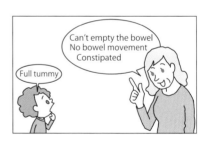

George： Shall I ask mom to give you an enema? She gives it to me when I have a bellyache.

Emma： Thank you, George. If the medicine doesn't work, will you ask your mother about the enema?

George： OK. Why can't you poop?

Emma： Maybe I didn't eat enough vegetables. Vegetables include a lot of fiber, which helps empty the bowels.

George： Mom always tells me to eat vegetables. Why didn't you eat a lot of vegetables?

Emma： I have had a toothache for a few days.

George： That's terrible. Grandma, you see a dentist, don't you?

Emma： Yes. I have an appointment this afternoon.

George： Poor grandma. I don't like the dentist. Aren't you afraid of dentists?

Emma： No way. They fix our tooth troubles!

George： I hate the sound when they are working on my teeth.

Emma： I always imagine that dwarfs are working in my mouth making noise. 5

George： Dwarfs are working in your mouth?

Emma： It is only my imagination, but it is fun.

George： I'll cross my fingers.

Emma visits the dentist, and a dental hygienist (DH) is checking her teeth. 10
Emmaは歯科医を受診し、歯科衛生士 (DH) がEmmaの歯を確認している。

DH： Good afternoon, Ms. Yamahara. My name is Hirata and I'm a dental hygienist.

Emma： Hello, Dr. Hirata.

DH： I'm sorry, but I'm not a doctor nor a dentist but a dental hygienist. 15

Emma： Oh, both you and a dentist take care of my teeth, don't you?

DH： That's true. Dentists' main role is treatment and dental hygienists' is prevention.

Emma： I see. I've also heard of a dental technologist. What do they do?

DH： They make and fix dentures. 20

Emma： I understand. The dentist explained to me that the cause of my toothache was periodontal disease. The best way to take care of this seems to be to remove dental calculus and plaque.

DH： That's right. I'm in charge of that care. Look in the mirror. You see the brown line on the bottom of your teeth. That's dental calculus. Let me recline the chair so that I can remove it. 25

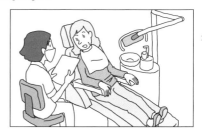

The DH scales the dental calculus. 30

DH： Please relax now. I'll return the chair to the original position, so please rinse your mouth.

Emma： Uh-huh.

Emma rinses her mouth a few times.

DH： Let me recline the chair once more to check how it is.

The dental hygienist checks Emma's teeth.

DH： Perfect. I've finished now. Please wait a little longer and let the dentist check.

Exercise 1. **Indicate True or False based on the dialog.**

会話文の内容に合っていれば T、合っていなければ F と記入しなさい。

( ) 1. Emma went to see a doctor because she was constipated.

( ) 2. George is given an enema when he has a bellyache.

( ) 3. Dwarfs are working in Emma's mouth and are making noise.

( ) 4. Emma had dental calculus removed.

Exercise 2. **Fill in the blanks of the following DH's report with words from the word list.**

次の歯科衛生士の記録の空所を語群の語で埋めなさい。

Emma understands the cause of her (1.   ). She was interested in the difference among a (2.   ), DH, and dental technologist. She learned the difference between (3.   ) and dental plaque and the importance of (4.   ) them.

Word list: dentist, dental calculus, removing, toothache

Anatomy and Physiology   Digestive System

Medical Terminology

accessory organ	付属器官	jejunum	空腸
alimentary canal	消化管	large intestine	大腸
anal canal	肛門管	liver	肝臓
anus	肛門	mastication	咀嚼
ascending colon	上行結腸	nutrient	栄養
bile	胆汁	oral cavity	口腔
cecum	盲腸	pancreas	膵臓
descending colon	下行結腸	pharynx	咽頭
digest	消化する	rectum	直腸
duodenum	十二指腸	ridge	尾根、隆起部
enzyme	酵素	salivary gland	唾液腺
esophagus	食道	sigmoid colon	S状結腸
feces	大便	small intestine	小腸
fold	くぼみ、谷の屈曲部	stomach	胃
gallbladder	胆嚢	tongue	舌
gastrointestinal tract		transverse colon	横行結腸
	消化管		
ileum	回腸		

Reading Comprehension

Based on the text below, please answer the following questions.

1. What does the digestive system involve besides the digestive tract?

2. What does the digestive system do after it breaks down food we eat?

3. What organs are included in the small intestine?

4. How long is the small intestine?

5. What are the accessory organs of the digestive system?

6. What is the main function of the liver?

7. How long is the large intestine?

8. Into where is bile released to dissolve fat?

The digestive system consists of the digestive tract, otherwise known as the alimentary canal or the gastrointestinal tract and accessory organs. The function of the digestive system is to breakdown food we eat into smaller components releasing their nutrients to be absorbed into the body.

The digestive tract is composed of a long tube of organs that runs from the mouth to the anus. It includes the oral cavity, pharynx, the esophagus, stomach, small intestine (duodenum, jejunum, and ileum), and large intestine (cecum, ascending colon, transverse colon, descending colon, sigmoid colon, and rectum). The accessory organs of the digestive system, such as the tongue, salivary glands, pancreas, liver, and gallbladder, work in coordination with the digestive tract.

Upon entering the mouth, food is chopped into smaller pieces by mastication before it is pushed into the pharynx, and then the esophagus, by the tongue and other muscles. The esophagus connects to the stomach, where food is stored as it is digested by enzymes. The small intestine, a 6 to 7 m long, tube-like organ, is located inferior to the stomach, and consists of a surface having many ridges and folds. These ridges and folds increase the efficiency of digestion and the absorption of nutrients. The final stage of digestion involves the large intestine. With a length of about 1.5 m and sitting inferior to the stomach, the large intestine extends all the way to the anus and serves to absorb water and break down waste to extract small amounts of nutrients. The waste (feces) in the large intestine exits the body through the anal canal.

The main function of the liver as an accessory organ of the digestive system is the production of bile that is stored and concentrated in the gallbladder, a pear-shaped organ under the right lobe of the liver. At meal time, bile is released into the duodenum to help dissolve fat into fluid content. The pancreas lies horizontally behind the bottom of the stomach and also makes enzymes to aid digestion.

Figure 1. 消化器系に関して、空所1〜18に適する語を英語で答えなさい。

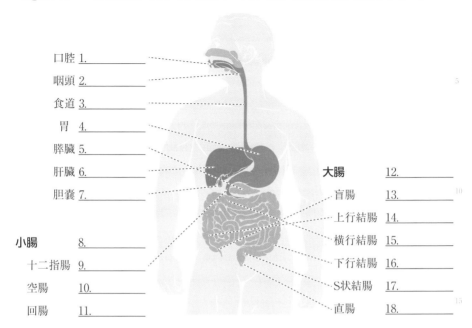

口腔 1. _____

咽頭 2. _____

食道 3. _____

胃 4. _____

膵臓 5. _____

肝臓 6. _____

胆嚢 7. _____

小腸 8. _____

十二指腸 9. _____

空腸 10. _____

回腸 11. _____

大腸 12. _____

盲腸 13. _____

上行結腸 14. _____

横行結腸 15. _____

下行結腸 16. _____

S状結腸 17. _____

直腸 18. _____

Exercise 1. 本文の要約となるように下の語群より適語を選び、空所を補充しなさい。

消化器系の機能は、食べたものを細分化し、食物の栄養が身体に吸収されるようにするための①_____と、②_____のような、消化の助けとなる酵素を作り出す付属器官より成り立っており、両者は互いに協調している。咀嚼によって小さくされた食物は、咽頭に送られ、③_____へ押し出されたのち、胃で貯えられ、④_____によって消化され、その後小腸へ送られる。小腸の壁にあるひだは消化を促進し、栄養を吸収する。消化の最終段階は肛門へと伸びる⑤_____で、そこでは水分を吸収し、少量の栄養分を絞り取る。消化器の付属器官である⑥_____は、胆汁の生成を司り、胆汁は⑦_____に貯えられ、濃縮された後、食事の際、脂肪を溶かすために⑧_____に放出される。

語群：胆嚢、肝臓、食道、酵素、十二指腸、膵臓、大腸、消化管

Exercise 2.　次の文章が本文の内容に合っているなら T を、合っていなければ F をそれぞれ記入しなさい。

(　) 1.　The goal of the digestive system is to breakdown waste into smaller pieces for the body to absorb the nutrients.

(　) 2.　An accessory organ is shaped like a long tube that runs from the mouth to the anus.

(　) 3.　The pancreas lies next to the stomach and stores bile produced by the liver.

(　) 4.　Mastication pushes food into the pharynx and conveys it into the esophagus.

(　) 5.　The small intestine is located under the stomach and is designed to absorb nutrients.

(　) 6.　The large intestine serves to absorb only water.

Unit

4

The Blood
【血液】

本課の ねらい	Dialog	貧血や管理栄養士に関する表現が使える。
	Anatomy and Physiology	血液の構成物と働きに関する英語表現を理解する。

4

Dialog   Anemia and Registered Dietitians

Medical Terminology

anemia	貧血	dizzy	めまいがする
bottle-feed	人工栄養で育てる	physician	内科医
breast-feed	母乳で育てる	registered dietitian	管理栄養士
dizziness	めまい		

Reading Comprehension

Based on the dialog below, please answer the following questions.

1. How long did Kay sleep well last night?
2. Why does Kay get up during the night?
3. How was Kay feeling when she was asked how she was by Ryuta?
4. Why did Ryuta look at Kay's nail color?
5. What did Kay's blood test results show?
6. What advice did the doctor give Kay?
7. According to the registered dietitian, what is helpful for those who suffer from some kinds of anemia?
8. How much iron is necessary per day for a breast-feeding female?

Kay (29 years old) is talking with her husband, Ryuta (31 years old), about her slight headache and dizziness after the birth of her child. Kay (29歳) は産後の軽い頭痛とめまいについて夫のRyuta (31歳) と話している。

Kay： Thank you Ryuta. Hadn't Naomi cried all night long?

Ryuta： She sometimes woke up but did not cry at all. Have you slept well?

Kay： Yes. I had a sound sleep for a few hours.

Ryuta： That's good. You must get up to breast-feed Naomi during the night. If she were bottle-fed, I could have helped you more.

Kay： Bottle-feeding is one option when my breasts can't produce enough milk, but I think it's lucky that I can nourish Naomi with my breast milk. You know it takes more time to prepare bottled milk.

Ryuta： Yes. We must keep a feeding bottle clean. We also have to prepare milk with boiled water and cool it down to a good temperature. But I can help you with that.

Kay： Oh, you gave me some time to sleep today. I am very grateful. I thank you.

Ryuta： It's my pleasure. How is your headache and dizziness?

Kay： I feel much better. But I still feel dizzy and tired.

Ryuta： You still look pale. I think you'd better see a doctor.

Kay： Don't you think it's natural to get tired from giving birth and taking care of a baby?

Ryuta： You also had to start a new life in a different country because of my relocation.

Kay： But my grandparents and mom help me a lot and everything is convenient here.

Ryuta： Let me see your nails.

Kay： I know you like my colorful nail polish but I don't have time to wear that.

Ryuta： No. I don't mean that. I want to see your actual nail color.

Kay： Oh, the color of my nails is whiter than before. Don't you think so?

Ryuta： It surely is. You might have anemia. You should see a doctor tomorrow.

Kay： OK. I will.

Kay is consulting with a registered dietitian (RD) because the physician diagnosed that her symptoms are caused by anemia and advised her to consult with an RD. 内科医にKayの症状は貧血によると診断され、管理栄養士に相談するように言われたので、KayはRDに相談している。

4

RD： According to the results of your blood test, your hemoglobin level was a little lower than the preferred level, which is between 11.5 g/dL and 14.5 g/dL.

Kay： Yes. Mine was 9.8 g/dL. The doctor told me to consult with a registered dietitian first instead of taking medication.

RD： A good diet is very helpful for those who suffer from some kinds of anemia.

Kay： I think I could get more iron from food.

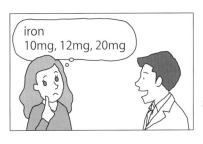

RD： That's right. They say that adult males should get 10 mg of iron per day and adult females should get more. Can you guess how much they need?

Kay： Hmm. If it is 10 mg for a man... is it 13 mg or 14 mg for a woman?

RD： That's close! 12 mg of iron are necessary for women per day. But you are breast-feeding. A breast-feeding female should have at least 20 mg of iron per day.

Kay： I eat spinach pretty often, but I don't like liver. What else contains lots of iron?

RD： Well, look at the first page of this booklet.

Kay： I didn't know green laver, Jew's-ear and clams have so much iron. Oh, iron in spinach is not as high as in parsley.

RD： If we eat the same amount of parsley as spinach, parsley has a lot more iron than spinach. But I think you wouldn't eat so much parsley.

Kay： I see.

RD： It's difficult to get enough nutrients from only a few kinds of food. Look at the rest of the pages in the booklet and choose a variety of food.

Food		iron in 100 g
green laver (dried)	アオノリ(乾)	77.0 mg
Jew's-ear (dried)	キクラゲ(乾)	35.2 mg
Japanese little neck clam (boiled)	アサリ(水煮)	29.7 mg
sardine (boiled and dried)	イワシ(煮干し)	18.0 mg
pork liver (uncooked)	豚レバー(生)	13.0 mg
hen's egg yolk (uncooked)	卵黄(生)	6.0 mg
parsley (uncooked)	パセリ(生)	7.5 mg
spinach (uncooked)	ホウレンソウ(生)	2.0 mg

食品成分データベース、文部科学省、https://fooddb.mext.go.jp/　2019.10.4閲覧

Exercise 1.　**Indicate True or False based on the dialog.**
会話文の内容に合っていればT、合っていなければFと記入しなさい。

( ) 1.　Bottle-feeding takes more time to prepare milk for babies.

( ) 2.　If she chose bottle-feeding, Ryuta could have helped Kay more.

( ) 3.　Ryuta does not like Kay's colorful nail polish.

( ) 4.　Iron in parsley is less than that in spinach.

Exercise 2.　**Fill in the blanks of the following RD's report with words from the word list.**
栄養士の記録の空所を語群の語で埋めなさい。

The (1.　) in Kay's blood was slightly lower than the preferred level. She understood

(2.　) females should take more iron than other women and the kinds of food that include much (3.　). She will choose a (4.　) of food for her good diet.

Word list： iron, hemoglobin, variety, breast-feeding

Anatomy and Physiology　The Blood

4

Medical Terminology

blood clot	血栓	lymph	リンパ(液)
blood vessel	血管	lymphatic vessel	リンパ管
capillary	毛細血管	pH (potential of hydrogen)	
carbon dioxide	二酸化炭素		水素イオン指数
cholesterol	コレステロール	plasma	血漿
clot	凝固させる	platelet	血小板
coagulation	凝固(物)	protein	タンパク質
erythrocyte	赤血球	prothrombin	プロトロンビン
fibrinogen	フィブリノゲン	red blood cell	赤血球
hemoglobin	ヘモグロビン	serum	血清
infection	感染	subclavian vein	鎖骨下静脈
inflammation	炎症	triglyceride	中性脂肪
interstitial fluid	間質液	white blood cell	白血球
leukocyte	白血球		

Reading Comprehension

Based on the text below, please answer the following questions.

1. How is blood related to body temperature?
2. What pH value is regarded as being healthy?
3. What kind of solid elements are there in blood?
4. How do leukocytes serve to maintain our health?
5. What is plasma made of?
6. Which is in larger ratio, the solid or liquid part of blood?
7. What includes platelets, fibrinogen and prothrombin?

8.   Into where does some of the fluid in the tissues flow?

Blood is a specialized fluid that circulates throughout the entire body.   The main functions of blood are as follows: transporting oxygen and nutrients to cells; protecting the body against infection and inflammation; regulating body temperature; maintaining a healthy pH value (around 7.4); maintaining the fluid content of the body; and forming blood clots (coagulation) to prevent excess blood loss.

The constituents of blood are solids and liquid. The solid parts of blood contain erythrocytes or red blood cells (RBCs), leukocytes or white blood cells (WBCs), and platelets. The liquid part, called plasma, is made of water, salts, and protein.

As its name implies, RBCs look red because they contain a large quantity of hemoglobin. RBCs deliver oxygen from lungs to organs and tissues, and they also help remove carbon dioxide (CO_2) from the body. WBCs are an important part of the immune system as they help protect the body from infections. Platelets help the blood clotting process—coagulation. These three solids make up 45-50% of the total blood volume.

The rest (50-55%) of the blood is liquid, called plasma. The main component of plasma is serum and the remaining parts include fibrinogen and prothrombin, which are involved in blood clotting. Various substances such as cholesterol, sugar, and triglycerides are dissolved in plasma and are carried throughout the body.

Some of the blood cells and fluid flow into the capillaries (the smallest type of blood vessel) and then into tissues. The fluid in the tissues is called interstitial fluid or tissue fluid. Some of the interstitial fluid flows into lymphatic vessels, resulting in lymph and returns to the circulatory system through the subclavian veins (refer to Unit 5).

Figure 1. 血液の成分に関して、空所に適切な英語を記入しなさい。

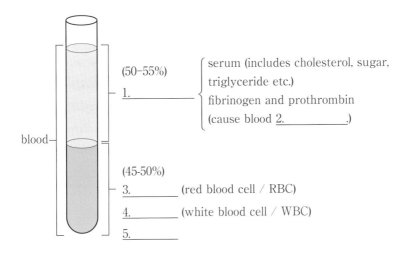

serum (includes cholesterol, sugar, triglyceride etc.)
fibrinogen and prothrombin
(cause blood 2._____.)

4

Exercise 1. 本文の要約となるように下の語群より適語を選び、空所を補充しなさい。

血液の主な機能は酸素や栄養素の運搬、①_____、体温調節、pH維持、体液量維持、止血である。血液の構成要素の半分弱が固体で、残りが液体である。前者はヘモグロビンを含み、酸素の運搬と二酸化炭素の排出を担う②_____と、①に関わる白血球、そして血液凝固に関係する③_____である。後者は④_____と呼ばれ、主な構成要素は⑤_____で、残りはフィブリノゲンやプロトロンビンといった血液凝固因子が含まれる。血液中の血球や液体は毛細血管へ、そして組織へと流れる。組織に含まれる液体は⑥_____と呼ばれ、一部は⑦_____に流れ、⑧_____を経て循環器系へと戻ってくる。

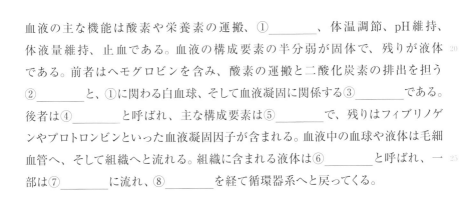

語群：間質液、血漿、鎖骨下静脈、赤血球、血小板、血清、リンパ管、感染予防

Exercise 2.　次の文章が本文の内容に合っているようなら T を、合っていなけれ
ば F を記入しなさい。

( ) 1.　The leukocytes protect the body from infections.

( ) 2.　The pH of the blood kept at 7.4 should be regarded as being abnormal.

( ) 3.　Only the platelets serve to stop bleeding by coagulation.

( ) 4.　The hemoglobin in erythrocytes carries oxygen to the lungs.

( ) 5.　The plasma is made of water, salts and protein.

( ) 6.　The interstitial fluid is called lymph.

Unit

The Circulatory System
【循環器系】

本課の ねらい	Dialog	心肺蘇生法、AED、胸部レントゲンや診療放射線技師に関する表現が使える。
	Anatomy and Physiology	循環器の各部位と循環の順に関する英語表現を理解する。

5

Dialog CPR and Radiological Technologists

Medical Terminology

AED (automated external defibrillator)		diagnose	診断する
	自動体外式除細動器	inhale	吸い込む
artificial ventilation	人工呼吸	radiation therapy	放射線治療
chest compression	心臓マッサージ	radiological technologist	
chest X-ray	胸部レントゲン		放射線技師
chin	あご先	tuberculosis	結核
CPR (cardiopulmonary resuscitation)			
	心肺蘇生		

Reading Comprehension

Based on the dialog below, please answer the following questions.

1. How often does Ryuta have a chance to practice CPR training at his company?
2. Has Ryuta ever performed the chest compression and AED in real life?
3. If we find an unconscious person, what should we do first?
4. When we face someone unconscious and if we cannot find anyone around us, what should we do?
5. How should we perform artificial ventilation?
6. What does AED stand for?
7. What are the radiological technologists' jobs?
8. What is the purpose of chest X-rays?

Ryuta (31 years old) and Kay (29 years old) are looking at a neighbor's circular notice and talking about CPR training. Ryuta（31歳）とKay（29歳）は町内で心肺蘇生の研修会が開かれるという回覧板を見て話し合っている。

5　Ryuta：　Here is the neighbor's circular informing us of a community meeting.

　　Kay：　　What is the purpose of the meeting?

　　Ryuta：　It seems to be regarding CPR training.

　　Kay：　　I want to learn about chest compression and AED.

　　Ryuta：　I have the opportunity to practice it at my company almost every year.

10　Kay：　　Then you can perform it if any of our family members has a heart attack.

　　Ryuta：　I've never thought of performing it in a real situation in my life.

　　Kay：　　But you may have to use it for me, and I would have to use it for you if you had such trouble.

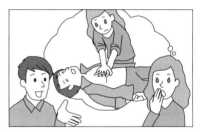

15　Ryuta：　Yes. To check if I am conscious, pat my shoulders and call my name or ask, "Are you OK?"

　　Kay：　　Where should I put my hands to perform chest compression?

20　Ryuta：　Just on the center of my chest. Place one of your hands on the top of the other and put both hands in the middle of the chest.

　　Kay：　　Press the center of your chest with both hands overlapping. How deep and fast should I press?

25　Ryuta：　About 5 cm at a rate of 100 times per minute. After pressing 30 times, you must provide artificial ventilation twice by exhaling air into my mouth while pinching my nose with your fingers.

　　Kay：　　You mean, 30 compressions and 2 mouth-to-mouth exhalings.

　　Ryuta：　Right. You should repeat this cycle until an ambulance arrives. If

30　　　　　　there's an AED, it's effective. I've forgotten what an AED stands for.

　　Kay：　　Here, it is written on the circular—automated external defibrillator.

Ryuta： Yes. Though it gives us audio guidance, I think you should learn how to use it.

Kay： Sure. I'll add my name to the list of participants. Shall we go together?

Ryuta： I'm sorry, I have to go to the hospital for a medical checkup on that day.

Ryuta is having a chest X-ray during his annual medical checkup. Ryutaは毎年の定期健診で胸部レントゲン撮影を受けている。(RT: radiological technologist)

5

RT： Hello, Mr. Yamahara. I'm a radiological technologist.

Ryuta： Yes. Only radiological technologists can take X-rays, right?

RT： Well, except for doctors, that's true.

Ryuta： I see. X-rays are an essential tool for doctors' diagnoses, aren't they?

RT： That's true. Radiation therapy is also crucial for patients with cancer.

Ryuta： Your job is very important in many ways.

RT： I take pride in my work. By the way, you are going to have a chest X-ray today?

Ryuta： Oh, I'm sorry I've wasted your time.

RT： That's OK. I'm glad you understand our job. Chest X-rays are not new to you, are they?

Ryuta： Of course not. I've had many chest X-rays since my high school days. They can detect tuberculosis, right?

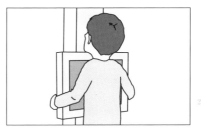

RT： That might be the main pur-pose, however, chest X-rays can find other diseases of the lungs and the heart.

Ryuta： Really? That's useful.

RT： OK. Would you stand here and put your chin on this? Then, put out your arms to hold the machine, please.

Ryuta： Like this?

RT： Very good. Please take a deep breath and hold it. I'll step out of the room.

Ryuta inhales deeply and holds it.

RT： Mr. Yamahara, relax now. That's it.

Ryuta： Thank you very much. I hope the results turn out well.

Exercise 1.　**Indicate True or False based on the dialog.**

会話文の内容に合っていればT、合っていなければFと記入しなさい。

( ) 1.　Ryuta and Kay signed up for the community meeting for the CPR training.

( ) 2.　Kay knows how to do chest compression.

( ) 3.　Ryuta has never attended the CPR training.

( ) 4.　Radiological technologists and doctors can take X-rays.

( ) 5.　Ryuta laid down to take a chest X-ray.

Exercise 2.　**Ryuta explains about the CPR and RT's job to Kay. Fill in the blanks with words from the list.**

RyutaがCPRとRTの仕事についてKayに説明している。空所を語群の語で埋めなさい。

CPR includes chest (1.　　), AED and artificial (2.　　). Radiological technologists not only take X-rays but also give radiation (3.　　). Chest X-rays detect diseases of the (4.　) as well as the diseases of the lungs.

Word list： heart, ventilation, therapy, compression

Anatomy and Physiology   **The Circulatory System**

Medical Terminology

aorta	大動脈	pulmonary circulation	
arterial	動脈の		肺循環
atrium	心房 (複数形は atria)	pulmonary vein	肺静脈
cardiovascular system		superior vena cava	
	心臓血管系		上大静脈 (複数形は superior venae cavae)
inferior vena cava	下大静脈 (複数形は inferior venae cavae)	systemic circulation	
			体循環
lymph node	リンパ節	venous blood	静脈血
lymphatic system	リンパ系	ventricle	心室
oxygenate	酸素化する	venule	細静脈
pulmonary artery	肺動脈		

5

Reading Comprehension

Based on the text below, please answer the following questions.

1. What is the core organ in the circulatory system?
2. What two circulation processes comprise the circulatory system?
3. Which part of the heart receives oxygen-poor blood and sends it to the lungs?
4. Which of the four chambers in the heart does the oxygenated blood pass through after it leaves the left atrium?
5. What is the smallest of the blood vessels?
6. What do large veins ultimately form?
7. Why is the lymphatic system closely related to the circulatory system?
8. What is the major difference between the lymphatic system and the circulatory system?

The circulatory system is a double system that consists of the heart and two functionally distinct circulations—the pulmonary and the systemic circulation. The heart is the key organ in the circulatory system, and it is divided into four chambers: two atria and two ventricles. The heart serves as a double pump that sends blood to the lungs (the pulmonary circulation) or to the rest of the body (the systemic circulation).

In pulmonary circulation, the right ventricle receives poorly oxygenated blood (venous blood) from the right atrium. And then it contracts and pumps the oxygen-poor blood to the lung through the pulmonary arteries enriching the blood with oxygen. The pulmonary veins return the oxygenated blood to the left atrium, from which it is sent to the left ventricle.

The path of the systemic circulation is between the heart and the rest of the body (excluding the lungs). After traveling through pulmonary circulation, oxygen-rich blood in the left ventricle leaves the heart via the aorta. More specifically, the contraction of the left ventricle of the heart forces the oxygenated blood (arterial blood) into the aorta. Large arteries branch off from the aorta to supply arterial blood to different areas of the body. Eventually, the small arterial vessels branch into capillaries. Then, the capillaries join together into venules, which in turn merge into increasingly large veins. Ultimately, those large veins form two core veins: the superior and inferior venae cavae.

The lymphatic system consists of lymphatic vessels and lymph nodes. The lymphatic vessels with lymph nodes lie just outside of the veins and the lymphatic system is closely related to the circulatory system. The lymph is drained into the subclavian vein near the heart, where it mixes with the venous blood. The main difference in the lymphatic system compared to the cardiovascular system is that the lymph goes in one direction towards the heart, while the blood circulates starting from the heart and returning to the heart.

Figure 1.   血液の循環に関して、空所1〜3に適する英語を答えなさい。

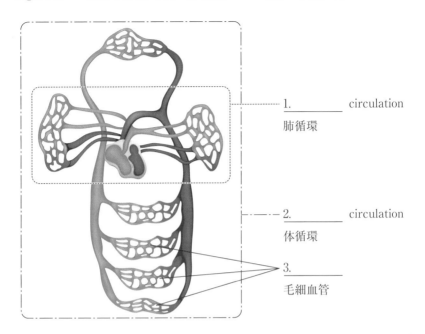

1. _____ circulation
肺循環

2. _____ circulation
体循環

3. _____
毛細血管

5

10

15

Figure 2.   心臓に関して、空所1〜9に適する語を英語で答えなさい。

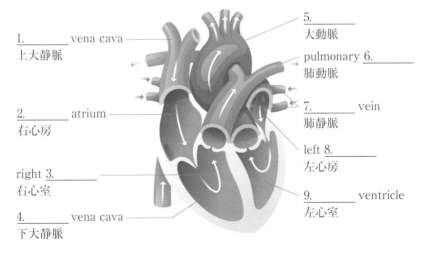

1. _____ vena cava
上大静脈

2. _____ atrium
右心房

right 3. _____
右心室

4. _____ vena cava
下大静脈

5. _____
大動脈

pulmonary 6. _____
肺動脈

7. _____ vein
肺静脈

left 8. _____
左心房

9. _____ ventricle
左心室

20

25

30

Exercise 1.　本文の要約となるように下の語群より適語を選び、空所を補充しなさい。

　　循環器系はポンプの機能を果たす心臓と循環（①_____・②_____）という2つのシステムから成る。①は心臓の右心房から取り入れた酸素の乏しい血液（静脈血）が③_____の収縮により④_____へ送られた後、肺で酸素の多い血液（動脈血）となり、肺静脈を経て⑤_____へ戻り、その後⑥_____へ送られるシステムである。

　　②では、その動脈血が⑥の収縮により⑦_____、そして分岐した動脈を経て、組織の毛細血管へと供給される。毛細血管は⑧_____へと集まり、その後大きな静脈へと合流し、最終的に中核となる2本の静脈（上・下大静脈）を形成する。

　　リンパ系はリンパ管と⑨_____から成り、⑩_____に沿って走行している。最終的にリンパ液は心臓近くの鎖骨下静脈に排出される。リンパ系が心臓に向かって一方向で走っているのに対し、循環器系は心臓から出発し心臓へと循環する。

> 語群：大動脈、静脈、肺動脈、細静脈、リンパ節、右心室、左心室、左心房、
> 　　　肺循環、体循環

Exercise 2.　次の文章が本文の内容に合っているなら T を、合っていなければ F をそれぞれ記入しなさい。

（　）1.　The venous blood is oxygenated in the heart.

（　）2.　The heart has two chambers.

（　）3.　The blood to the lungs from the right ventricle is arterial blood.

（　）4.　The large artery branches to the aorta and circulates.

（　）5.　The blood comes back from the whole body to the left atrium.

（　）6.　The lymph is mixed with the blood near the heart.

Unit 6
The Respiratory System
【呼吸器系】

本課の ねらい	Dialog	在宅酸素療法や社会福祉士に関する表現が使える。
	Anatomy and Physiology	呼吸器の各部位と空気の流れに関する英語表現を理解する。

Dialog   Home Oxygen Therapy and Certified Social Workers

Medical Terminology

care manager	介護支援専門員	humidifier	加湿器
certified social worker	社会福祉士	nasal cannula	鼻腔カニューレ
compressed oxygen	圧縮酸素	oxygen concentrator	酸素濃縮器
concentrate	濃縮する	oxygen cylinder	酸素ボンベ
flowmeter	流量計	oxygen therapy	酸素療法
HOT (home oxygen therapy)	在宅酸素療法	public health nurse	保健師

Reading Comprehension

Based on the dialog below, please answer the following questions.

1. What is the role of an oxygen concentrator?
2. Why is a nasal cannula important?
3. What does Shinji put in a small cart when he goes out?
4. How often does Shinji go out?
5. How does Shinji prepare his meals?
6. What is annoying Shinji about visitting his sister's family?
7. What do people with oxygen cylinders do at a gathering?
8. Why did Shinji decide to join the gathering?

Kenzo (80 years old) visits his friend Shinji Ibe (78 years old) who is having home oxygen therapy (HOT). 在宅酸素療法 (HOT) をしているShinji(78歳)宅を、Kenzo(80歳)が訪問している。

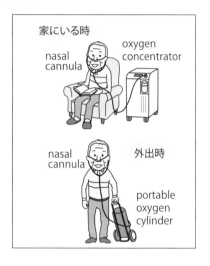

家にいる時
nasal cannula
oxygen concentrator

nasal cannula
外出時
portable oxygen cylinder

Kenzo： Hello. Long time no see. You look good.

Shinji： How kind of you to come see me! I'm doing well because of this device called oxygen concentrator.

Kenzo： What does it do?

Shinji： It concentrates the oxygen out of the air.

Kenzo： So, you can breathe in oxygen as far as this tube reaches.

Shinji： This tube is called a nasal cannula.

Kenzo： What are these attached to the device?

Shinji： These are a flowmeter and a humidifier, and they show the oxygen flow and the water level of the humidifier.

Kenzo： It seems important. What do you do when you go out?

Shinji： I can use a portable oxygen cylinder.

Kenzo： It is small but isn't it heavy to carry?

Shinji： I can move it around in this small cart.

Kenzo： I see. Is liquid oxygen filled in this tank?

Shinji： No, it is compressed oxygen. Some people like liquid oxygen and the same volume lasts longer, but it is more difficult to use.

Kenzo： So, you can go out freely with a portable oxygen cylinder.

Shinji： That's true, though I don't feel like going out except to see a doctor.

Kenzo： Don't you enjoy traveling these days? You used to enjoy driving, didn't you?

Shinji： I usually stay at home since becoming unable to drive. It is bothersome to go out.

Kenzo： I know. But I often enjoy a bus tour with my wife. It's convenient.

Shinji： I'm afraid I will have some trouble because of the oxygen therapy.

Kenzo： Have you talked to a public health nurse or a care manager about your situation?

Shinji： Well, a certified social worker will visit me tomorrow morning.

Kenzo： That's good. I hope you can talk about going out to see other people then.

A certified social worker (CSW), Fukuhira visits Shinji and invites him to a gathering of people having HOT. 社会福祉士（CSW）のFukuhiraがShinjiを訪ね、HOTを受けている人の集いに誘っている。

CSW： Good morning, Mr. Ibe. I'm Fukuhira, a certified social worker of this city.

Shinji： Nice to meet you, Mr. Fukuhira.

CSW： Are you having any problems in your daily life?

Shinji： No. I can do everything by myself. As for meals, my sister brings them every day.

CSW： That's great. Don't you join your sister's family for dinner?

Shinji： It's annoying to carry a portable cylinder to visit them. So, I ask her to deliver my meals.

CSW： You can go and see a doctor regularly by yourself, right?

Shinji： Yes. I take a bus to the clinic by myself. Other than that, I don't go out.

CSW： I see. Why don't you come to a gathering of many people with oxygen cylinders?

Shinji： What do they do there?

CSW： They talk, sing, play games, and other such things.

Shinji： I'm sorry but I'm not so interested.

CSW： There will be newcomers who have just started life with HOT. Would you share your story with them?

Shinji： Talking about my story? It is neither attractive nor special.

CSW： It is good to tell them that life with HOT is not a special one.

Shinji： My life with HOT is not special at all. I live a normal life with the devices.

CSW： They are worried whether or not they can manage HOT correctly. Would you tell them what you are doing?

Shinji： I only check the oxygen flow and water level of the humidifier every day.

CSW： That's important. Would you tell them how simple that is? They will be encouraged if you show that you can live without any problem having HOT.

Shinji： If I can be of help to them... Where is the gathering held?

CSW： It's in the city hospital near the clinic you usually visit.

Shinji： Great. I can go by bus, then.

CSW： That's wonderful. We'll gather on the 7th floor at 10 o'clock next Tuesday.

Shinji： OK. I will go and tell them how I feel much better with HOT.

CSW： I am so grateful. We look forward to it. If you have any question, please call this number.

Exercise 1. Indicate True or False based on the dialog.

会話文の内容に合っていればT、合っていなければFと記入しなさい。

( ) 1. Kenzo visits Shinji every other day.

( ) 2. Shinji's portable oxygen cylinder is filled with liquid oxygen.

( ) 3. Shinji used to enjoy driving.

( ) 4. Shinji is going to the city hospital to join the gathering at 10 o'clock next Tuesday.

Exercise 2. Fill in the blanks of the following CSW's report with words from the word list.

次のCSWの記録の空所を語群の語で埋めなさい。

Mr. Ibe seemed to welcome my (1.   ) though he does not like going out. He can live without any problem with the help of his sister bringing (2.   ). He did not show any (3.   ) in the gathering, however, he showed his will to help people who need (4.   ). I hope it will turn out to be a good (5.   ) for him to go out.

Word list：interest, HOT, opportunity, meals, visit

Anatomy and Physiology   The Respiratory System

Medical Terminology

alveolar	肺胞の	glottis	声門
alveolus	肺胞 (複数形は alveoli)	larynx	喉頭
bronchiole	細気管支	moisten	湿らせる
bronchus	気管支 (複数形は bronchi)	mucous	粘液の
		nasal cavity	鼻腔
cartilage	軟骨	olfactory mucosa	嗅粘膜
cartilaginous	軟骨性の	trachea	気管
chemical receptor	化学受容体	vocal fold	声帯
gland	分泌腺		

Reading Comprehension

Based on the text below, please answer the following questions.

1. What is the respiratory system composed of?
2. What is the respiratory system designed to do?
3. What do the vocal folds and the space between them make?
4. What enters the lungs along with the blood vessels?
5. What is the structural basis for the main function of the respiratory system?

6. What are the two respiratory organs that never close?
7. What are the respiratory passages mostly covered by?
8. What function does the olfactory mucosa serve?

The respiratory system consists of the lungs and the respiratory passages (respiratory tracts) and it is responsible for the exchange of oxygen and carbon dioxide. Air enters the body through the nasal and oral cavities and passes through the pharynx into the larynx. In the center of the larynx lies the glottis, which is composed of vocal folds and the spaces between them. After exiting the larynx, air enters the trachea. The trachea divides into the left and right main bronchi in the thorax. Each bronchus enters a lung and continues to branch into smaller passages, called bronchioles.

Blood vessels also enter the lungs with the bronchi; the blood vessels come into intimate contact with alveoli which are the terminal units of the bronchioles. This intimate relationship between pulmonary capillaries and alveolar air spaces is the structural basis for the main function of the respiratory system. Both the capillaries and alveoli have extremely thin walls, allowing the oxygen to pass from the alveoli to the blood.

The larynx and the trachea are rigid tubes that never close because the larynx is protected on the outside by thick cartilage and the trachea has a series of C-shaped cartilage in its wall.

The respiratory passages are mostly covered by a mucous film that is produced by glands within the wall of the respiratory passages. This mucous film has several functions, such as trapping small particles when air is inhaled, moistening the air, and keeping the underlying tissues moist. Other components of the respiratory system also serve different functions. For example, the olfactory mucosa in the nasal cavity serves as a chemical receptor for smell, and the larynx serves in making sounds.

Figure 1. 呼吸器に関して、空所に適切な英語、あるいは日本語を記入しなさい。

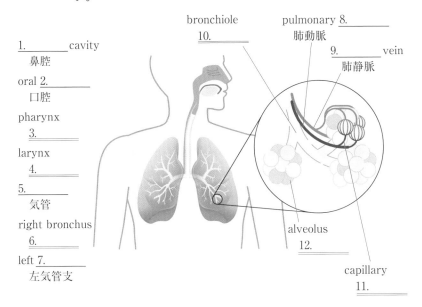

1. _____ cavity
鼻腔

oral 2. _____
口腔

pharynx
3. _____

larynx
4. _____

5. _____
気管

right bronchus
6. _____

left 7. _____
左気管支

bronchiole
10. _____

pulmonary 8. _____
肺動脈

9. _____ vein
肺静脈

alveolus
12. _____

capillary
11. _____

Exercise 1. 本文の要約となるように下の語群より適語を選び、空所を補充しなさい。

　呼吸器系は肺と①_____で成り立っており、空気は鼻腔・口腔を経て咽頭、喉頭、そして声門、気管、左右の②_____へ送られる。②は血管と共に両肺に入り、③_____と呼ばれる細い管へと分岐する。③の末端は④_____と呼ばれ、呼吸器系の構造の基礎は肺の毛細血管と④の空間が密に接する関係にある。厚い軟骨で守られた喉頭と、C字型の連続した⑤_____を持つ気管は共に決して塞がらない。これらは呼吸器官の壁から分泌される⑥_____で覆われており、この膜は呼吸の際、微粒子を捕えたり、空気や⑦_____を湿らせるといった作用がある。その他、呼吸器系の機能としては、嗅粘膜が匂いのための⑧_____になったり、喉頭には音声を作る働きがある。

語群：化学受容体、粘液、肺胞、組織、気管、気管支、細気管支、軟骨、気道

Exercise 2.   呼吸器系の働きについて、空欄を埋めなさい。

1. Exchange of _____ and _____ _____ .

2. Air is brought into the body, through nasal and oral cavities → _____
   → larynx, glottis → _____ → right and left bronchi → _____
   → _____ (the terminal)

3. The oxygen passes from the alveoli to the blood because both the _____
   and alveoli have extremely _____ walls.

4. The _____ film that is produced by glands within the wall of the
   passage serves to trap small particles in the inhaled air, to moisten the
   _____ , and to keep the underlying _____ moist.

5. The olfactory _____ serves as a chemical receptor for _____ .

6. The _____ in the larynx serves in making _____ .

Unit 7

The Urinary System
【泌尿器系】

本課の ねらい	Dialog	脱水、頻尿、膀胱炎や臨床検査技師に関する表現が使える。
	Anatomy and Physiology	泌尿器の各部位に関する英語表現を理解する。

Dialog   Dehydration and Medical Technologists

Medical Terminology

antibiotic	抗生物質	dehydration	脱水（症状）
bacteria	細菌（複数形は bacterium)	gynecology	婦人科
cerebral infarction	脳梗塞	medical technologist	臨床検査技師 (MT)
cultivate	培養する	urologist	泌尿器科医
cystitis	膀胱炎	urology	泌尿器科
dehydrate	脱水する		

Reading Comprehension

Based on the dialog below, please answer the following questions.

1. Why didn't Susie drink a glass of water even though she was sweating?

2. What will happen to how we feel thirsty when we get old?

3. What would happen if we didn't drink enough water?

4. What did Ichiro suggest to Susie about drinking 1.2 liters of water a day?

5. What kind of trouble does Susie have when she tries to leave the house?

6. After Susie talked with Ichiro, what rule did she make regarding water intake?

7. Why did Susie feel that she might be dehydrated?

8. Why do MTs cultivate the urine which is collected?

Susie (77 years old) is talking about water intake with her grandson Ichiro (26 years old). Susie（77歳）と孫のIchiro（26歳）が水分摂取について話し合っている。

Susie：　It's so hot today! I only took out the garbage and I am sweating all over.

Ichiro：　Grandma, would you like a glass of cold water?

Susie：　No, thank you. I would have to go to the restroom again. It's annoying to go to the restroom so often.

Ichiro：　Oh, that's why you don't drink much water?

Susie：　Well, I do not feel thirsty. If I felt thirsty, I would drink water.

Ichiro：　I've heard that people feel less thirsty when they get older.

Susie：　Then, we old people don't have to drink as much as young people do, do we?

Ichiro：　I don't think that's right. Drinking enough water is important to prevent dehydration.

Susie：　I often hear about that. But I urinate only a little every time I use the restroom. I drink less and urinate less. Don't you think I'm safe from dehydration?

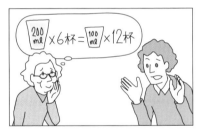

Ichiro：　No way. Though you may think your water balance is good, I've read in the paper that we need at least 1.2 liters of water a day to get rid of waste from the body.

Susie：　Really? More than a liter is too much for me!

Ichiro：　You don't have to drink it all at one time. If we don't drink enough, our blood will thicken, and could cause problems like a cerebral infarction.

Susie：　That's terrible.

Ichiro：　Instead of drinking 200 mL of water 6 times, how about drinking 100 mL of water 12 times?

Susie：　That sounds easier, though I'm afraid I would go to the restroom more often.

Ichiro： Think positively. Going to the restroom would be good exercise for you! By the way, one of my friends, Satoshi, will visit me next week.

Susie： That's fantastic. I really want to see him.

Ichiro's friend Satoshi, a medical technologist (MT), is talking to Susie. Ichiro の友人で臨床検査技師 (MT) である Satoshi は Susie と話している。

Susie： Hi, Satoshi. It has been a long time. How have you been doing?

Satoshi： Hi, Susie. I'm doing very well. How are you?

Susie： Not bad but getting older is troublesome in every way.

Satoshi： In every way? What troubles you, for example?

Susie： When I go out, I feel sluggish in putting shoes on or locking the door. At the supermarket, it takes time to read an ingredient list and to pay the cashier. And I sometimes have to stop packing the groceries to go to the restroom.

Satoshi： You go to the restroom during your grocery packing?

Susie： Yes. After Ichiro told me to drink more water, I made a rule to drink a half glass of water every hour.

Satoshi： That's important. How often do you go to the restroom?

Susie： I usually go to the restroom maybe 10 times a day, but from this morning, I go every thirty minutes. I urinate so often that I might be dehydrated.

Satoshi： Don't worry about dehydration at this point. What's more worrisome is cystitis.

Susie： I've heard women suffer from that disease more than men.

Satoshi： It is not a fatal disease if you treat it properly with antibiotics.

Susie： Then I'm going to a drugstore now.

Satoshi： Wait. You'd better see a doctor. Only a doctor can diagnose your problem, not me.

Susie： OK. What doctor do you think I should see, a physician or a urologist?

Satoshi： I recommend you go to a urology clinic. A gynecology clinic is another option.

Susie： OK. As an MT, would you tell me what examination I should take?

Satoshi： A patient usually has only a urine test in such cases.

Susie： I know I should collect urine from mid-stream, right?

Satoshi： That's right. And the urine is analyzed and cultivated by MTs.

Susie： Why do you cultivate?

Satoshi： It is hard to see a small number of bacteria, so we increase their numbers to see them well.

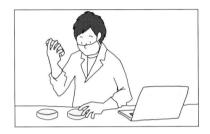

Susie： Then, do I have to wait before I take any medicine for the cultivation process to complete?

Satoshi： No. A doctor usually prescribes common medicine before a definite diagnosis.

Susie： Oh, please excuse me, I need to go to the restroom.

Exercise 1.   **Indicate True or False based on the dialog.**

会話文の内容に合っていればT、合っていなければFと記入しなさい。

( ) 1.   Susie drinks enough water for her hydration after talking with Ichiro.

( ) 2.   We need 0.5 liters of water a day to excrete waste from our bodies.

( ) 3.   Satoshi was worried about Susie's dehydration.

( ) 4.   Satoshi advised Susie to go to the drug store to buy medicine.

Exercise 2.   **Fill in the blanks of Satoshi's memo to Ichiro with words from the word list.**

次のSatoshiのIchiroへのメモの空所を語群の語で埋めなさい。

Susie follows your (1.   ) and seems to start drinking enough water. She might

(2.   ) that the reason she goes to the restroom more than ever is just because she

started drinking more (3.   ), however, the frequency of (4.   ) seems unusual, so I told her to go to see a (5.   ).

Word list: doctor, advice, think, urination, water

Anatomy and Physiology   **The Urinary System**

Medical Terminology

bladder	膀胱	renal artery	腎動脈
Bowman's capsule		renal corpuscle	腎小体
	ボウマン嚢	renal cortex	腎皮質
calyx	腎杯 (複数形は calyces)	renal glomerulus	腎糸球体 (複数形は renal glomeruli)
filtrate	濾液		
kidney	腎臓	renal medulla	腎髄質
nephron	ネフロン	renal pelvis	腎盂、腎盤
nerve	神経	renal tubule	尿細管
peritoneum	腹膜	renal vein	腎静脈
purify	浄化する	ureter	尿管
reabsorb	再吸収する	urethra	尿道

7

Reading Comprehension

Based on the text below, please answer the following questions.

1. What does the urinary system consist of?
2. What do the kidneys do to blood?
3. How big are the kidneys?
4. What are two elements that compose the renal medulla?
5. What does a Bowman's capsule surround?
6. What does the nephron consist of?
7. What does the bladder do with urine?
8. What is the difference between a man's and woman's urethras?

The urinary system consists of two kidneys, two ureters, the bladder and the urethra. The renal veins, the renal arteries and nerves enter the kidneys which lie behind the peritoneum. The kidneys have three functions. First, they purify blood. When blood passes through the kidneys, waste products are removed and passed on to the bladder. Second, the kidneys help control the potential of hydrogen (pH) of the internal environment. Third, the kidneys reabsorb water, salt and sugar elements in the blood for reuse in the body.

Each kidney is about 10 to 12 cm long, roughly the size of a large fist, and has an outer rim, the renal cortex, and an inner region, the renal medulla. The renal medulla is composed of many calyces and renal pelvises. The renal cortex has multiple renal glomeruli, each of which is surrounded by a Bowman's capsule. A unit made of a renal glomerulus and a Bowman's capsule is called the renal corpuscle. This unit and the renal tubule constitute the nephron. More than one million nephrons are in each kidney. The Bowman's capsule, a cup-like sack, collects the filtrate and empties it into the renal tubule where necessary substances are reabsorbed from the filtrate to make urine. The urine is sent to the ureters through the renal pelvises and then to the bladder to be held temporarily until it is excreted through the urethra.

Each ureter is a muscular tube about 25 cm long, and the bladder has the size and shape of a pear. The urethra measures about 3.8 cm long in a woman and 20 cm in a man. Women are more likely than men to get a bladder infection because the urethra is much shorter in a woman than in a man.

Figure 1. 泌尿器系に関して、空所に適切な英語、あるいは日本語を記入しな
さい。

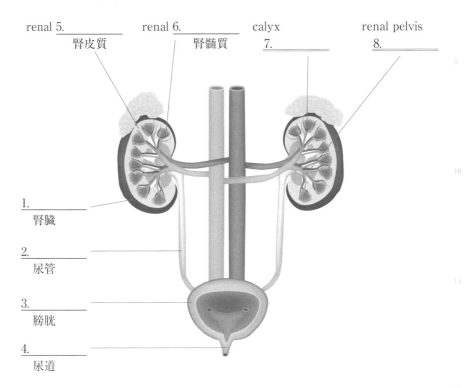

renal 5. _____
腎皮質

renal 6. _____
腎髄質

calyx
7. _____

renal pelvis
8. _____

1. _____
腎臓

2. _____
尿管

3. _____
膀胱

4. _____
尿道

Figure 2. ネフロンの構成に関して、空所に適切な英語、あるいは日本語を記
入しなさい。

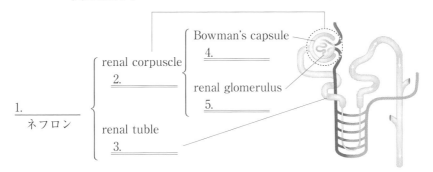

1. _____
ネフロン

renal corpuscle
2. _____

renal tuble
3. _____

Bowman's capsule
4. _____

renal glomerulus
5. _____

Exercise 1.　本文の要約となるように下の語群より適語を選び、空所を補充しなさい。

　　泌尿器系は①_____、②_____、③_____、④_____で成り立っている。腎臓へは腎動脈、腎静脈、神経が出入りしており、その内側を⑤_____、外縁を⑥_____という。⑤を構成するのは主に⑦_____と⑧_____であり、⑥には100万以上の⑨_____が存在する。⑨は⑩_____を⑪_____が覆うような形態の⑫_____とそれに続く尿細管で形成され尿の生成を行っている。⑨で生成された尿は、⑦、⑧を経て尿管を通り、膀胱で一時的に貯えられ、膀胱の下部から出ている尿道を通って排尿される。

> 語群：腎盂、腎小体、腎髄質、腎臓、腎杯、腎皮質、糸球体、尿管、ネフロン、尿道、ボウマン嚢、膀胱

Exercise 2.　腎臓の機能に関して、下の語群の中から適語を選び（　　　　）を埋めなさい。その際、必要に応じて形を変えなさい。

1. Kidneys purify (　　). Waste products are (　　) and passed on to the (　　).
2. Kidneys help control the (　　) in the body.
3. In the renal tubule, the substances that are necessary for the body, (　　), (　　) and sugar in the blood, are absorbed from the (　　).
4. In the urinary system, the urine is sent to the (　　) through the (　　) and then to the bladder.
5. Women have much shorter (　　) than men do.

> 語群：bladder, blood, filtrate, pH, remove, renal pelvis, salt, ureters, urethra, water

Unit

The Central Nervous System
【中枢神経系】

本課の ねらい	Dialog	認知症、長谷川式認知症スケールや臨床心理士に関する表現が使える。
	Anatomy and Physiology	中枢神経の各部位に関する英語表現を理解する。

Dialog　Dementia and Clinical Psychologists

Medical Terminology

Alzheimer's disease	アルツハイマー病	HHS (U.S. Department of Health and Human Services)	
clinical psychologist	臨床心理士		アメリカ合衆国保健福祉省
cognitive function test	認知機能検査		
dementia	認知症	MCI (mild cognitive impairment)	
forgetfulness	物忘れ		軽度認知障害
HDS-R (Hasegawa's Dementia Scale-Revised)	改訂長谷川式認知症スケール	neurologist	神経内科医

Reading Comprehension

Based on the dialog below, please answer the following questions.

1. What was Kenzo looking for?

2. How did Kenzo find his glasses?

3. What does Susie often forget?

4. What did Susie forget in her thirties?

5. What does MCI stand for?

6. Why did Kenzo and Susie go to see a doctor?

7. How well did Kenzo do on the subtraction test?

8. Using a hint, what word could Kenzo come up with?

Kenzo (80 years old) and Susie (77 years old) are worried about their recent forgetfulness. Kenzo（80歳）とSusie（77歳）は最近の物忘れを心配している。

Kenzo： Good morning, Susie. Do you know where my glasses are?

Susie： Glasses? Didn't you put them on the washstand?

Kenzo： Oh, thank you. I found them there. Why do you know I left them there?

Susie： Well, you've often left them on the washstand after you have washed your face.

Kenzo： That's true. I often forget my glasses and keys.

Susie： I often leave my cellphone at home when I go out.

Kenzo： Yes. When I call you while you are out, your phone often rings in the house.

Susie： I'm sorry. Don't you think we have both forgotten things too often recently?

Kenzo： Is it natural or the beginning of Alzheimer's disease?

Susie： I can't recall the name of a mild condition of forgetfulness.

Kenzo： You mean MCI, or mild cognitive impairment?

Susie： That's it. You see I can't recall things.

Kenzo： It is natural. If we could remember everything, I think we would be able to get a perfect score on every exam.

Susie： Yes. We are not geniuses. But we never forgot the name of a superstar.

Kenzo： You once forgot our wedding anniversary, didn't you? You were in your thirties.

Susie： You remember very well! It's sure that you don't have Alzheimer's disease.

Kenzo： Let's look it up online. I found a site about MCI. Look, Susie.

Susie： It is by the U.S. Department of Health and Human Services. It must be reliable.

Kenzo： Memory problems are caused not only by Alzheimer's disease but also by aging, emotional problems, MCI and other types of dementia.

Susie： OK, but is MCI different from memory problems caused by aging?

Kenzo： They say, memory problems caused by MCI are more severe than those caused by normal aging and milder than those caused by Alzheimer's.

Susie： Are you sure our cases are normal and not MCI?

Kenzo： It says we should see a doctor early when we have unusual memory problems.

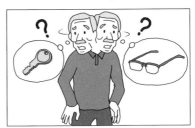

Kenzo and Susie saw a neurologist and were told to get a cognitive function test from a clinical psychologist (CP). Susie has finished the test named HDS-R (Hasegawa's Dementia Scale-Revised) and Kenzo is taking it now. KenzoとSusieは神経内科医を受診し臨床心理士（CP）の認知機能検査を受けるように言われた。SusieがHDS-R（長谷川式認知症スケール）と呼ばれる検査を終え今度はKenzoが受けている。

CP： Let's go to the next question. Can you subtract 7 from 100?

Kenzo： That's simple. 93.

CP： That's right. Please continue subtracting 7 from the answer.

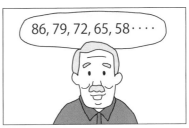

Kenzo： 86, 79, 72, 65, 58...

CP： Thank you. Now, I will say some numbers. Would you say the numbers in reverse order? Six, eight, two.

Kenzo： Two, eight, six.

CP： Good. Next, nine, two, five, three.

Kenzo： Three, five, two,... I can't recall what the first number was.

CP： OK. Next question. Tell me the three words I asked you to memorize a little while ago?

Kenzo： Cherry blossom, train and ...

CP： It was an animal.

Kenzo： Ah, a cat.

CP： Good. I will show you five things. Please name the items after I hide
　　　 them.

The CP shows a watch, a key, a pack of cigarettes, a coin and a pen slowly
naming them one by one and hides them.

Kenzo： A coin, a key, a pen, a watch and cigarettes.

CP： Great! Here comes the last question: Please name as many vegetables
　　　 as you can.

Kenzo： Radish, cucumber, carrot, onion, potato, pumpkin, green pepper, egg-
　　　 plant, lettuce, cabbage, leek, lotus, spinach, beansprout, and green
　　　 bean...

CP： You named a lot. That's all for the test. The doctor will explain your
　　　 results later. Would you sit in the waiting room for a while?

Kenzo： Thank you very much.

Exercise 1.　Indicate True or False based on the dialog.
　　　　　　会話文の内容に合っていればT、合っていなければFと記入しなさい。

( ) 1.　Recently, Kenzo and Susie have both forgotten things.

( ) 2.　Memory problems are caused by Alzheimer's disease and other factors
　　　　including aging.

( ) 3.　Kenzo and Susie were told to take a test by a CP.

( ) 4.　"Tomato" was one of Kenzo's answers to the last question by the CP.

**Exercise 2.　Fill in the blanks of the following CP's report with words from the
　　　　　　word list.**
　　　　　　次のCPの記録の空所を語群の語で埋めなさい。

Kenzo had no problem in doing (1.　), however he failed in the backward repeating
of four (2.　). As for "the delayed recall test," he could tell (3.　) names without a
hint and one with a hint. After watching five things, he could (4.　) all five successfully.
Lastly, he named 15 (5.　).

Word list： numbers, vegetables, plants, subtraction, recall, two, three

Anatomy and Physiology　**The Central Nervous System**

Medical Terminology

ataxia	運動失調症	gray matter	灰白質
axon	軸索	medulla oblongata	
blood pressure	血圧		延髄
brain	脳	mesencephalon	中脳
brain stem	脳幹	nerve cell	神経細胞
cardiac	心臓の	nervous system	神経系
cell body	細胞体	neuron	ニューロン、神経単位
cerebellum	小脳	organism	有機体、生物体
cerebral cortex	大脳皮質	PNS (peripheral nervous system)	
cerebrum	大脳		末梢神経系
CNS (central nervous system)		pons	橋
	中枢神経系	respiration	呼吸
cross-section	断面	spinal cord	脊髄
dendrite	樹状突起	synapse	シナプス
diencephalon	間脳	white matter	白質

Reading Comprehension

Based on the text below, please answer the following questions.

1. What is the main functional cell in the nervous system called?
2. What are the two projections that a neuron has?
3. What are the two categories of the nervous system?
4. What does gray matter of the CNS contain?
5. What are the three regions of the brain?
6. What purpose does the cerebral cortex serve?
7. How does the cerebellum function?
8. What does the brain stem connect?

Nerves are distributed throughout the human organism, forming the nervous system, which plays a vital role in determining how information is transmitted throughout the body. The main functional cell in the nervous system is the nerve cell or neuron. Each neuron has three elements: the cell body, short projections called dendrites and an elongated projection named axon. Basically, a message or signal is passed from one neuron to another at the synapse between the axon of one neuron and the dendrites of the next neuron.

The nervous system can be divided into the central nervous system (CNS) and the peripheral nervous system (PNS). The CNS includes all the structures within the brain and spinal cord, and the PNS involves all the nerves that exist outside of the CNS. This unit deals with the CNS and unit 9 addresses the PNS. The tissues of the CNS are divided into gray matter that contains a high density of cell bodies, and white matter which is composed of a large number of axons.

The brain, a component of the CNS can be divided into three regions: the cerebrum, cerebellum, and brain stem. The cerebrum is the largest region and has gray matter on the surface called the cerebral cortex. The cerebral cortex, which is more developed in higher animals, is the center of most activities, sensations, and mental processes such as thought, intelligence, memory and language. The cerebellum is located below the cerebrum. It controls the balance and movements of the body. When someone has a disease in the cerebellum, it is not life threatening but the person may have ataxia and walk as if he or she were drunk.

The brain stem is the collective name for the diencephalon, mesencephalon, pons and medulla oblongata, which is located below the cerebrum and in front of the cerebellum. The brain stem connects the cerebrum and the spinal cord. This part of the brain is vital for the transfer of information between the cerebrum and the spinal cord, and it regulates essential functions such as respiration, cardiac activity, blood pressure and other functions.

The spinal cord, which continues from the brain stem, has gray matter in the center shaped like an "H" in a cross-section and white matter surrounds the gray matter.

Figure 1. ニューロン(神経単位) に関して、空所1〜3に適する英語を答えなさい。

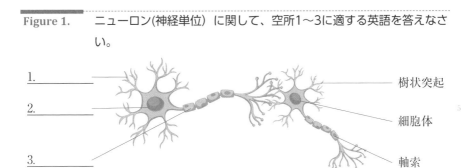

1. _____
2. _____
3. _____

樹状突起

細胞体

軸索

Figure 2. 中枢神経系に関して、空所に適切な英語、あるいは日本語を記入しなさい。

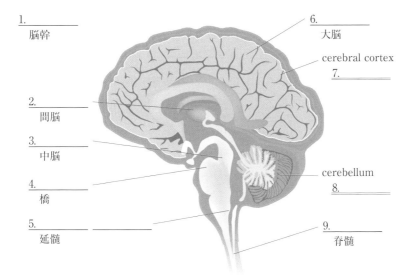

1. _____
   脳幹

2. _____
   間脳

3. _____
   中脳

4. _____
   橋

5. _____
   延髄

6. _____
   大脳

cerebral cortex
7. _____

cerebellum
8. _____

9. _____
   脊髄

Exercise 1.　本文の要約となるように、下の語群から適語を選び空所に記入しなさい。

　　①_____と②_____から成る神経系の機能の要は③_____（神経単位）である。

　　③は④_____、樹状突起、⑤_____という3つの要素を持っている。情報伝達はシグナル（活動電位）が一つのニューロンの⑤と次のニューロンの樹状突起の間で受け渡しが起こり実行される。①は脳や脊髄を含み、その組織は④が密集する灰白質と多くの⑤より成る白質からできている。

　　脳と脊髄で中枢神経系を成す。脳の3分野は⑥_____、⑦_____、⑧_____であり、⑥の表面には灰白質の⑨_____がある。⑨は高等動物においてより発達しており、行動、感覚、知的精神活動の中心である。大脳の下に位置する⑦は身体の運動や平衡感覚を制御する。⑧は間脳、⑩_____、⑪_____、⑫_____の集合体を表す名称で、大脳と脊髄を結んでいる、この間の情報伝達において重要な部位で、呼吸、血圧等、生命維持機能の中心である。脳幹に続く脊髄の断面を見ると、中央のH字状の灰白質の周りを白質が囲む構造をしている。

> 語群：大脳、中脳、小脳、大脳皮質、脳幹、橋（脳橋）、延髄、ニューロン、中枢神経系、末梢神経系、軸索、細胞体

Exercise 2.　本文の内容に合っていれば T を、合っていなければ F を記入しなさい。

(　)1.　The brain and the spinal cord make up the central nervous system.

(　)2.　The area filled with axons in the central nervous system is white matter.

(　)3.　The axon is one of the components of the dendrites and the nerve cell body.

(　)4.　The cerebral cortex serves to control the sensations and respiration.

( ) 5. The brainstem includes the cerebellum.

( ) 6. A person that has a problem in the cerebrum may develop ataxia.

( ) 7. The spinal cord has gray matter that is shaped like an "H" in the center of a cross-section.

Unit 9
The Peripheral Nervous System
【末梢神経系】

本課の ねらい	Dialog	脱臼、神経麻痺や理学療法士に関する表現が使える。
	Anatomy and Physiology	末梢神経の分類と働きに関する英語表現を理解する。

Dialog   Neuropathy and Physical Therapists

Medical Terminology

aerobic exercise	有酸素運動	dislocation	脱臼
complication	合併症 (通例この 意味では複数形)	fracture	骨折
diabetes	糖尿病	neuropathy	ニューロパシー、 神経障害
diabetic nephropathy	糖尿病性腎症	physical therapist	理学療法士 (PT)
diabetic neuropathy	糖尿病性神経障害	reduction	整復
diabetic retinopathy	糖尿病性網膜症	sling	三角巾(固定具)

Reading Comprehension

Based on the dialog below, please answer the following questions.

1. What did Kay hope to achieve by running?
2. What did Ryuta and Kay see and find when they were running?
3. What happened to Ryuta when he tried to find a cute dog?
4. Why did Ryuta think he may have a broken bone?
5. How did Ryuta get to the clinic with his dislocated shoulder?
6. For how long has Ryuta's shoulder been in a sling?
7. Why did Ryuta think that he felt difficulty moving his arm?
8. In total, how many times a day should Ryuta do the rehabilitation for his arm that the PT instructed?

Ryuta (31 years old) gets hurt while jogging with Kay (29 years old) and comes back to see an orthopedic surgeon. Ryuta（31歳）はKay（29歳）とジョギング中にケガをし、整形外科受診をしようと帰宅する。

5 Ryuta： It's a beautiful day, isn't it?

Kay：   It sure is. Would you run a little slower today?

Ryuta： Is it too fast? I'm running at a usual pace. Are you feeling OK?

Kay：   I am fine but I just heard on TV yesterday that it is better to run slowly as if we were walking.

10 Ryuta： I think it depends on what you hope to achieve by running. Slow running is good to burn body fat as aerobic exercise, whereas faster running is more effective at training the muscles.

Kay：   You are very knowledgeable. Then, I would like to run slowly.

Ryuta： OK. Let's run to enjoy the morning air. Look! The leaves are turning

15   red and yellow.

Kay：   Yes. There are acorns here and there.

Ryuta： You might bump into a passerby if you are looking downward. Be careful.

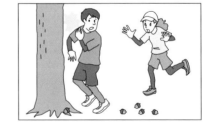

20 Kay：   OK. Oh, what a cute dog!

Ryuta： A dog! Where is it? Ow!

Kay：   Are you OK? Have you run straight into a tree?

Ryuta： It really hurts. I told you to be sure to look forward, but...

25 Kay：   Where is the pain?

Ryuta： I have an unusual pain in my right shoulder. I may have a broken bone. I can't move my right arm.

Kay：   Oh my god! Do you think you can walk home?

Ryuta： Why not. What I hurt is not legs or feet but my shoulder.

30

Ryuta's shoulder was diagnosed as dislocated and had reduction by a doctor. After keeping it in a sling for about three weeks, he visited the orthopedic clinic and is now talking to a PT (physical therapist). Ryutaの肩は脱臼と診断され医師による整復がなされた。約3週間、固定具で固定後、整形外科を受診し理学療法士と話している。

5

PT： The doctor told you that your bone was not damaged.

Ryuta： Yes, and he told me that there seemed to be only a little damage in other tissues around the bone.

PT： It was good that you didn't move your shoulder before you saw the doctor.

10

Ryuta： It was too painful to move the shoulder.

PT： I know. But some patients try to move their shoulders before they come here.

Ryuta： I must thank my wife for driving me here so I could hold my arm.

PT： It is your first time to have a dislocated shoulder, isn't it?

15

Ryuta： Yes. I've never experienced a bone fracture nor dislocation before.

PT： You are lucky. Some people experience shoulder dislocations several times.

Ryuta： Really? I don't want to have such an experience again.

PT： Nobody does. Your shoulder has been healing well for three weeks.

20

Ryuta： So, the next step is rehabilitation, isn't it?

PT： Yes. Your nerves were damaged a little, and your muscles got smaller.

Ryuta： Is it the so called neuropathy?

PT： Why do you know the term? You are the first patient who has known the word.

25

Ryuta： My father has diabetes and we learned about its complications.

PT： I see. Its three major complications are diabetic nephropathy, diabetic neuropathy and diabetic retinopathy. OK. Let's

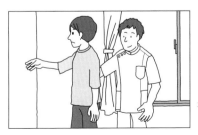

30

return to your case.

Ryuta：　I thought the reason why I have had a hard time moving was because I have not worked out much.

PT：　That's right. Your joints became stiff because you have not been using them much.

Ryuta：　OK and what kind of rehabilitation do I need?

PT：　First, stand facing the wall and raise your right arm horizontally in front of you touching the wall like this.

Ryuta：　Wow. I never thought it was so tough to raise to that level.

PT：　Go down slowly. OK. Turn to me and raise your arm to the right, up to shoulder height, along the wall. Don't raise your arm higher than shoulder level.

Ryuta：　It is hard too. How many times should I do this?

PT：　Thirty times is one set and please do the set twice a day.

Ryuta：　I see. When shall I visit again? It is difficult for me to come here on weekdays.

PT：　Then do this exercise at home until next Saturday unless you experience unusual pain.

Exercise 1.　**Indicate True or False based on the dialog.**

会話文の内容に合っていればT、合っていなければFと記入しなさい。

（　）1.　Ryuta knows more about running than Kay.

（　）2.　Ryuta could not walk for a while after the accident.

（　）3.　Regarding Ryuta's shoulder, his bones were not damaged.

（　）4.　If Ryuta's shoulder is painless, he will not see the PT until next Saturday.

Exercise 2.　**Fill in the blanks of the following PT's report with words from the word list.**

次のPTの記録の空所を語群の語で埋めなさい。

Ryuta started the (1.   ) of raising his arm forward and to the (2.   ) up to the height of his (3.   ) three weeks after the accident. It seemed to be (4.   ) to raise his arm, however, he will (5.   ) the directed set of exercise at home (6.   ) a day until the following Saturday.

Word list: hard, shoulder, side, twice, rehabilitation, continue

Anatomy and Physiology   The Peripheral Nervous System (PNS)

Medical Terminology

afferent	求心性の	parasympathetic nervous system	
antagonistic	拮抗の		副交感神経系
autonomic nervous system		sensory nerve	感覚神経
	自律神経系	somatic nervous system	
cranial nerve	脳神経		体性神経系
efferent	遠心性の	spinal nerve	脊髄神経
heart rate	心拍数	stimuli	刺激
impulse	インパルス	sympathetic nervous system	
metabolism	代謝		交感神経系
motor nerve	運動神経		

Reading Comprehension

Based on the text below, please answer the following questions.

1. What is the PNS made of?
2. What are the two nervous systems of the PNS on a functional basis?
3. What are the two subsidiary categories of the somatic nerves on a functional basis?
4. What is a difference between the sensory nerves and motor nerves?
5. What are the two subsidiary categories of the somatic nerves on a structural level?
6. How many pairs of cranial nerves are in the body?

7. How do autonomic nerves control the body?

8. What are the two autonomic nerves that work as an agonistic pair called?

The peripheral nervous system (PNS) is one of two components that composes the nervous system (the other one is the central nervous system, the CNS, studied in unit 8). The PNS consists of all nerves that exist outside the brain and spinal cord. The peripheral nervous system connects the CNS (made of the brain and spinal cord) to various parts of the body, serving as a communication pathway between them. On a functional basis, the PNS is divided into the somatic nervous system and the autonomic nervous system.

Functionally, the somatic nervous system can be further divided into sensory (afferent) and motor (efferent) nerves, depending on whether they bring information to the CNS or carry messages towards muscles, organs or other parts. More specifically, sensory nerves that receive information from external stimuli such as the senses of vision, hearing, taste, and smell, carry sensory information to the CNS, while motor nerves transmit impulses to contract muscles. In a structural level, the peripheral nerves are categorized into two separate segments: 12 pairs of cranial nerves are connected to the brain, whereas 31 pairs of spinal nerves are connected to the spinal cord.

Autonomic nerves control a wide range of systems within the body, regulating the cardiac and smooth muscle activities, endocrine gland secretions, and the metabolism of certain cells. Autonomic nerves are not generally under our conscious control but they serve many crucial functions such as the digestion of food and the maintenance of blood pressure. The autonomic nervous system is divided into an antagonistic pair of sympathetic and parasympathetic nervous systems. For example, the sympathetic nervous system triggers the body's automatic response to danger resulting in increasing the heart rate, raising the blood pressure and slowing digestion. On the other hand, the parasympathetic nervous system, for instance, slows the heart rate, lowers the blood pressure, and promotes digestion.

Figure 1. 末梢神経系に関して、空所に適する英語を答えなさい。

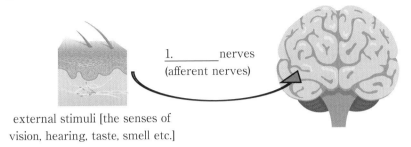

1.＿＿＿＿＿ nerves
(afferent nerves)

external stimuli [the senses of
vision, hearing, taste, smell etc.]

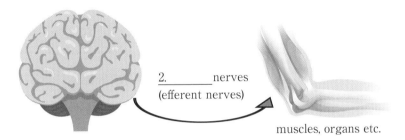

2.＿＿＿＿＿ nerves
(efferent nerves)

muscles, organs etc.

Figure 2. 自律神経に関して、空所1〜5に適する英語を答えなさい。

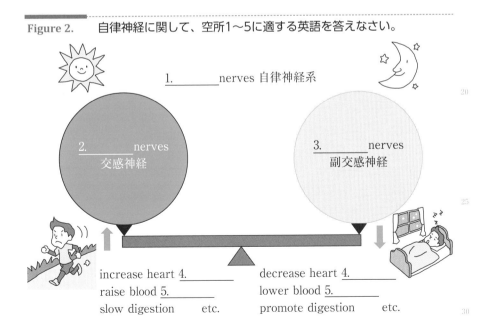

1.＿＿＿＿＿ nerves 自律神経系

2.＿＿＿＿＿ nerves
交感神経

3.＿＿＿＿＿ nerves
副交感神経

increase heart 4.＿＿＿＿＿   decrease heart 4.＿＿＿＿＿
raise blood 5.＿＿＿＿＿   lower blood 5.＿＿＿＿＿
slow digestion   etc.   promote digestion   etc.

Exercise 1.　本文の要約となるように、下の語群から適語を選び空所に記入しなさい。

中枢神経系と共に神経系を形成する末梢神経系は①_____と②_____の2種に分けられる。機能的にみると、①には視覚、聴覚、味覚のように中枢に信号を伝える③_____と、中枢から筋肉や器官、その他の部位へメッセージを伝える④_____に分類される。さらに構造的にみた場合、体性神経系は、脳につながる⑤_____と、脊髄につながる⑥_____に分別される。

②は⑦_____や平滑筋の調整、内分泌腺の分泌、特定の細胞の代謝といった広範な制御を行う。また、②によって、消化や血圧の維持のような重要な機能が⑧_____になされているが、これは自律神経系が相反する⑨_____と⑩_____の神経系に分かれているためで、⑨が心拍を高め血圧を上昇させるのに対し、⑩は心拍を遅くし、血圧を低下させる。

語群：脳神経、脊髄神経、運動神経、感覚神経、体性神経系、自律神経系、
　　　交感神経、副交感神経、無意識、心筋

Exercise 2.　末梢神経系の種類について、空所に適切な英語、日本語、また⑧には数字を記入しなさい。

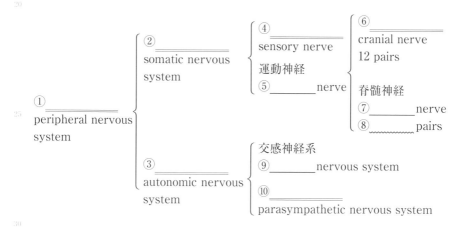

Unit

10

The Sensory System
【感覚器系】

本課の ねらい	Dialog	結膜炎、鍼治療や鍼灸師に関する表現が使える。
	Anatomy and Physiology	感覚器のうち目と耳の構造に関する英語表現を理解する。

Dialog　Allergic Conjunctivitis and Acupuncturists

Medical Terminology

acupuncture	鍼（治療）	itchiness	かゆみ
acupuncturist	鍼師	medical sheet	問診票
allergic	アレルギー性の	neuralgia	神経痛
allergy	アレルギー	ophthalmologist	眼科医
congest	充血する	pollen	花粉
conjunctivitis	結膜炎	rheumatoid arthritis	関節リウマチ
eczema	湿疹	sleeplessness	不眠
frozen shoulder	五十肩	white	白目
infectious	感染性の		

Reading Comprehension

Based on the dialog below, please answer the following questions.

1. How long has Emma had itchy eyes?

2. What does Emma think is the cause of her itchy eyes?

3. What did Ken tell Emma to do before her going to the ophthalmologist?

4. What did Emma's friend tell her about his pollen allergy?

5. For which disorders with pain does acupuncture seem to be effective?

6. What symptom does Emma think is the most problematic?

7. How fast does acupuncture work?

8. Why was Emma asked to show her tongue to the acupuncturist?

Ken (58 years old) worries about Emma's (54 years old) congested eyes and they are talking together. Ken (58歳)はEmma (54歳)の目が充血しているのを心配し、2人で話し合っている。

Ken： The whites of your eyes are red. Look in the mirror.

Emma： Oh, they're really red. My eyes have been so itchy for about two days.

Ken： Have you rubbed your eyelids because they were itchy?

Emma： My eyes were so itchy that I couldn't stop rubbing. It may be because of a pollen allergy.

Ken： Have you suffered from a pollen allergy before?

Emma： No. But according to the newspaper, anyone can get it all of a sudden.

Ken： I know. But isn't it out of season? My colleagues with pollen allergy aren't wearing masks lately.

Emma： I've heard that there are various kinds of pollen that affect people all year round.

Ken： That reminds me that my colleagues were complaining about cedar pollen.

Emma： You see? My allergy may be caused by the pollen of cypress or other plants.

Ken： Can't your problem be conjunctivitis caused by bacteria or viruses?

Emma： Oh dear! They are infectious, aren't they? Bob once had viral conjunctivitis.

Ken： Yes, I remember. The virus spreads so easily that he was suspended from school for a few days. We washed our hands countlessly at that time!

Emma： I must go to the ophthalmologist today.

Ken： Before you go out, wash your hands completely with soap.

Emma： Yes. We really learned how to wash hands at that time. Do you remember?

Ken： Leave it to me. First, wet our hands completely with water.

Emma： Second, apply soap to our hands. And third, rub our palms.

Ken： Fourth, rub the backs of our hands...and fifth, rub between the fingers.

Emma： Sixth, rub each thumb by holding it with the other hand.

Ken： Seventh, rub the fingertips of each hand against the palm of the other hand.

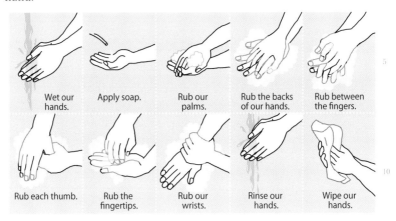

| Wet our hands. | Apply soap. | Rub our palms. | Rub the backs of our hands. | Rub between the fingers. |
| Rub each thumb. | Rub the fingertips. | Rub our wrists. | Rinse our hands. | Wipe our hands. |

Emma： Eighth, rub your wrists and ninth, rinse your hands under running water.

Ken： OK. Lastly wipe with a clean towel. Perfect. Don't touch your eyes, please.

10

Emma's eyes were diagnosed as allergic conjunctivitis. She wants to try acupuncture treatment and now she is talking with an acupuncturist (AP). Emmaの目はアレルギー性結膜炎と診断された。彼女は鍼治療を試そうと思い、鍼師 (AP) と話している。

AP： Come in please. Put your belongings in the basket there and have a seat here.

Emma： Yes. Thank you. Hello, Sir.

AP： Hello, Mrs. Yamahara. According to your medical sheet, your problem is allergic conjunctivitis, isn't it?

Emma： Yes. My friend told me that his pollen allergy has gotten better with acupuncture.

AP： That's wonderful! Acupuncture treatment is also effective for disorders with pains such as neuralgia, rheumatoid arthritis and frozen shoulder.

Emma： Acupuncture seems to be effective for diseases with pain, doesn't it?

AP： Pain is one of the symptoms patients most often complain about and acupuncture tends to ease their pain, however, dizziness or sleepless-ness are treated with acupuncture too.

Emma： I understand. I hope my itchiness will get better with acupuncture.

AP： Itchiness can also be serious. We also treat patients with eczema or conjunctivitis.

Emma： Then will my eyes stop being itchy with acupuncture?

AP： Many patients with conjuncti-vitis have recovered by using acupuncture.

Emma： I know the effect varies from person to person, but I believe it's worth trying.

AP： And please remember, it may take a while to work on any symptoms.

Emma： I understand. I know the effect appears slowly with eastern medicine compared to western medicine. How long will it take?

AP： Some patients feel the effect from the first time and others notice changes after several treatments.

Emma： I see. Will you do acupuncture for me?

AP： Sure. First, may I see your tongue?

Emma： Tongue? OK.

AP： The condition of the tongue gives us a lot of information about the patient.

Exercise 1.　**Indicate True or False based on the dialog.**

会話文の内容に合っていればT、合っていなければFと記入しなさい。

( ) 1.　Emma has once suffered from a pollen allergy.

( ) 2.　Bob was not able to go to school when he had viral conjunctivitis.

( ) 3.　It is not necessary for fingertips to be washed with soap to prevent the infection.

( ) 4.   Compared to western medicine, eastern medicine, such as acupuncture, tends to work slower.

Exercise 2.   **Fill in the blanks of the following AP's report with words on the
word list.**

次のAPの記録の空所を語群の語で埋めなさい。

Emma's problem is (1.   ) eyes and her condition was (2.   ) by an ophthalmologist as
allergic (3.   ). She understood the potential of (4.   ) and that the (5.   ) may be mild
and appear differently from person-to-person.

> Word list： acupuncture, itchy, conjunctivitis, diagnosed, effects

Anatomy and Physiology   **The Sensory System**

10

Medical Terminology

anterior chamber	前房	optic chiasm	視交叉
auditory area	聴覚野	optic nerve	視神経
cochlea	蝸牛	pupil	瞳孔
cochlear nerve	蝸牛神経	retina	網膜
cornea	角膜	spiral organ	ラセン器、コルチ器
external ear	外耳	stapes	アブミ骨
incus	キヌタ骨	temporal lobe	側頭葉
internal ear	内耳	tympanic membrane (eardrum)	
lens	水晶体		鼓膜
malleus	ツチ骨	visual area	視覚野
middle ear	中耳	vitreous body	硝子体
occipital lobe	後頭葉		

Reading Comprehension

Based on the text below, please answer the following questions.

1. What does the sensory system convert the stimuli to?
2. In which part of the body is the impulse interpreted as sensation?
3. What do eyes do after they perceive light and focus on objects?
4. Which part of the eyes converts the light stimulus to an impulse?
5. Where is the visual area located in the brain?
6. How many bones are there in the middle ear?
7. What organ receives a sound wave in the internal ear?
8. Where are the auditory areas located in the brain?

Sensory systems control our important senses including vision, hearing, touch, taste, smell and balance. We see with our eyes, hear and feel balance with our ears, taste with our tongue, smell with our nose, and feel pain in a damaged area of our body. However they are not felt as sensations until the information is transported as impulses to the brain. Namely, sensory organs receive many stimuli from inside and outside of the body and convert them to impulses which are interpreted as sensations in the brain.

The eyes are one of the smallest organs and their functions and structures are complex. Functionally, each eye constantly adjusts how much light it lets in, focuses on objects that are near and far, and constructs images that are promptly transmitted to the brain. The following process describes how we perceive and transmit light structurally. Light stimulus enters the cornea, anterior chamber, pupil, lens, vitreous body and retina of the eye, where it is converted to an impulse. The impulse is transmitted through the optic nerve and the optic chiasm to the visual areas of the brain. The visual area is located in the back of the brain in an area called the occipital lobes of the cerebral cortex. Visual disorders are usually caused by problems occurring in areas between the eye and the brain.

The ear is composed of three parts: the external ear, the middle ear and the internal ear. All three parts of the ear are crucial for detecting sound by working together to transfer sound from the external part through the middle and into the internal part of the ear. Also, ears help to maintain balance.

   This is how we detect a sound. A sound wave is gathered in the external ear, transmitted to the tympanic membrane (eardrum) and vibrates it. In the middle ear, the vibration is transmitted to the malleus, the incus and the stapes. In the internal ear, a sound wave is received in the spiral organ of the cochlea, then transmitted to the auditory area of the brain through the cochlear nerve. After all these steps are followed, a sound is recognized. The auditory areas are located at the sides of the brain in an area called the temporal lobes of the cerebral cortex.

Figure 1.   目に関して、空所に適切な英語、あるいは日本語を記入しなさい。

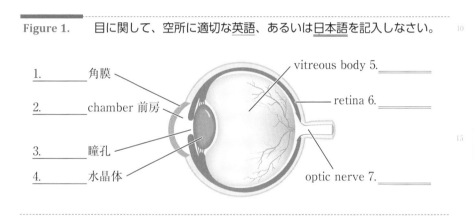

1._____ 角膜

2._____chamber 前房

3._____瞳孔

4._____水晶体

vitreous body 5._____

retina 6._____

optic nerve 7._____

Figure 2.   視覚の情報の伝わり方に関して、空所に適切な英語、あるいは日本語を記入しなさい。

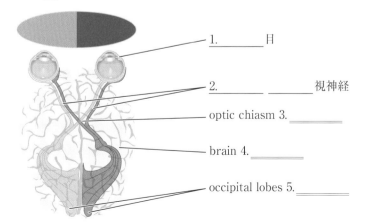

1._____目

2._____ _____視神経

optic chiasm 3._____

brain 4._____

occipital lobes 5._____

Figure 3. 耳に関して、空所に適切な英語、あるいは日本語を記入しなさい。

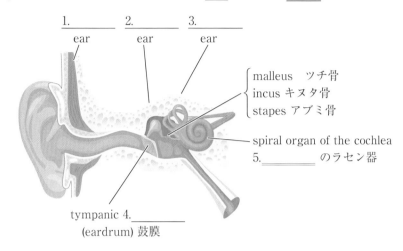

1. _____ ear
2. _____ ear
3. _____ ear

malleus　ツチ骨
incus キヌタ骨
stapes アブミ骨

spiral organ of the cochlea
5. _____ のラセン器

tympanic 4. _____
(eardrum) 鼓膜

Exercise 1. 本文の要約となるように下の語群より適語を選び、空所を補充しなさい。

　感覚器において、我々はさまざまな刺激を感受し、それを① _____ に変換した情報が脳へ伝えられ、感覚として感じられる。

　最小の器官の一つである目が司る視覚は、光の刺激が角膜、② _____ 、水晶体、硝子体を経て③ _____ で①に変換され、視神経と④ _____ を通じて脳の視覚野へと伝達される。視覚野は⑤ _____ に位置している。

　耳は音を感知し、⑥ _____ を取るための役割がある。聴覚は、外耳で集められた音波が⑦ _____ を振動させ、中耳(ツチ骨、キヌタ骨、⑧ _____)へ伝えられ、内耳の⑨ _____ にあるラセン器で受容され、蝸牛神経を経て大脳皮質の⑩ _____ で知覚される。

語群：側頭葉、後頭葉、鼓膜、蝸牛、網膜、瞳孔、視交叉、アブミ骨、インパルス、バランス

Exercise 2. 光刺激と音波の伝わり方について空所を補充し、日本語と英語でまとめましょう。

【光刺激】

日本語	光刺激 → 角膜 → ① ____ →
	② ____ → ③ ____ → 硝子体 →
	④ ____ → 視神経、⑤ ____ → 視覚野
英　語	light impulse → ⑥ ____ → anterior chamber →
	⑦ ____ → lens → ⑧ ____ →
	⑨ ____ → optic nerve, ⑩ ____ → visual area

【音波】

日本語	音波 → 外耳 → ① ____ （振動）→
	〔中耳：ツチ骨、② ____ 、アブミ骨〕→
	〔内耳：③ ____ 〕 → 蝸牛神経 → 聴覚分野
英　語	sound wave → external ear → ④ ____ (vibration) →
	〔middle ear: malleus, the incus, stapes〕→
	〔internal ear: ⑤ ____ 〕→ cochlea nerve → auditory area

10

Unit

11

The Skin
【皮膚】

本課の ねらい	Dialog	アトピー性皮膚炎、離乳食や保健師に関する表現が 使える。
	Anatomy and Physiology	皮膚の構造と働きに関する英語表現を理解する。

Dialog　**Atopic Dermatitis and Public Health Nurses**

Medical Terminology

atopic dermatitis	アトピー性皮膚炎	rash	湿疹
dermatologist	皮膚科医	scab	かさぶた
hormonal	ホルモンの	scaliness	ガサガサの状態
inheritance	遺伝	scratch	引っ掻く、引っ掻き
moisturizer	保湿剤		傷
predisposition	(ある種の病気にか かりやすい) 体質		

11

Reading Comprehension

Based on the dialog below, please answer the following questions.

1. When did small rashes appear on Naomi's cheeks?
2. What did Kay buy for Naomi to help prevent her from scratching her cheeks?
3. What skin problem does Ryuta not want Naomi to have growing up?
4. How does Kay feed milk to Naomi?
5. How long has Naomi had baby food?
6. What baby food was fed to Naomi after she got used to rice gruel?
7. When should Kay take her baby to see a dermatologist?
8. Why should mittens be taken off if Naomi doesn't scratch her rashes?

Ryuta (31 years old) is talking with Kay (29 years old) about their daughter Naomi's (4 months old) skin problems. Ryuta (31歳) はKay (29歳) と娘の Naomi (4か月) の皮膚の問題について話し合っている。

Ryuta： Kay, there's something strange on Naomi's cheeks. Did she scratch again?

Kay： No. Small rashes came out last week and now they have become scabs.

Ryuta： Oh, you are smiling at Dad, Naomi. They are not itchy, are they?

Kay： If she could tell me with words, it would be easier to know her problems.

Ryuta： Naomi, you will talk a lot soon, won't you?

Kay： She's in a good mood and cheerful. So, I don't think they are itchy.

Ryuta： Well, she might scratch her cheeks again. Wouldn't it be helpful to cut her nails?

Kay： I cut them, but her nails can still leave scratches.

Ryuta： Really? How about mittens? I've seen a baby wearing them.

Kay： What a coincidence! I just ordered them online yesterday.

Ryuta： Good for you! Do I need to wash her more gently when bathing her?

Kay： You wash and rinse her skin so gently that she always looks comfortable.

Ryuta： I had atopic dermatitis as a child and I don't want her to have it.

Kay： I agree. Her skin has been perfect except for the scratches and the current trouble.

Ryuta： OK. Isn't it better for her to see a dermatologist?

Kay： A public health nurse will visit us next week. I'll ask her about that.

Ryuta： OK. Oh, she's ready to cry. Good girl, Naomi. Are they itchy?

Kay： She must be hungry now. Wait a moment, Naomi. Dad will give you baby food.

Ryuta： Now I remember, you told me that she began baby food. Can I give it to her?

Kay： Sure. Here's rice gruel I cooked for her.

Ryuta：　Only this? What a poor meal! Can I give her eggs or fish?

Kay：　She just started baby food a week ago. She can't eat eggs or fish for a few weeks.

Ryuta：　Is that so? OK. Naomi, eat this. Look! She ate rice gruel. Is that all?

Kay：　Yes. I'll increase the portion little by little. Thank you, Ryuta. I'll breast-feed now.

A public health nurse (PHN) visits Kay to see how things are going with her baby. 保健師 (PHN) が赤ん坊との生活の様子を見るために Kay を訪問している。

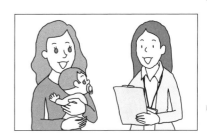

PHN：　Hi, how are you doing?

Kay：　Very well, thank you. Naomi is gaining weight favorably, and she started baby food two weeks ago as you advised me last month.

PHN：　That's good.

Kay：　About two weeks ago when she started baby food, she had rashes. Do they have something to do with the baby food?

PHN：　Did she start from a spoonful of rice gruel once a day?

Kay：　Yes. And I tried carrot paste yesterday. She doesn't have any problem eating.

PHN：　Let me see her cheeks. They have healed well. Some babies have rashes soon after their birth and until they are a few months old. They are said to be some hormonal effect.

Kay：　Are they atopic dermatitis? My husband had that trouble growing up.

PHN：　We cannot deny the inheritance of predisposition, however, her skin doesn't seem to have such a problem.

Kay：　Yes, her skin is beautiful now, but her cheeks looked terrible last week.

PHN：　Babies' skin tends to be dehydrated from two or three months old and if it gets rough to the touch, it's better to put cream on to prevent dryness and scaliness.

Kay：　Should I put in some bath salt for a baby taking a bath?

PHN： It's not necessary. It is important to keep her skin clean by washing softly and keep her skin moist by applying moisturizer.

Kay： I understand well. Keep her skin clean and moist.

PHN： Good. Even if you take care of her skin well and she has terrible rashes for a long period, then it may be a good idea to see a dermatologist.

Kay： I've put mittens on her hands so that she will not scratch her skin. Is it OK?

PHN： Well, mittens prevent babies from controlling their temperature through their hands. So, if Naomi doesn't scratch her rashes, mittens should be taken off.

Kay： I understand.

Exercise 1.　**Indicate True or False based on the dialog.**
会話文の内容に合っていればT、合っていなければFと記入しなさい。

(　) 1.　Ryuta bathes Naomi and she always looks comfortable.

(　) 2.　Naomi could have eggs as soon as she started to have rice gruel.

(　) 3.　Some babies have rashes soon after their birth because of their hormonal effect.

(　) 4.　Bath salt is important to keep the skin clean and moist.

Exercise 2.　**The following is the PHN's record about Naomi. Fill in the blanks with words from the list.**
次はNaomiについてのPHNの記録です。空所を語群の語で埋めなさい。

Naomi's parents are (1.　) about her rashes and scabs because of her father's atopic predisposition. Her skin (2.　) to be in good condition and her mother was advised to (3.　) her skin clean and to (4.　) moisturizer if it gets dehydrated. Her baby food phase is (5.　) smoothly and she will (6.　) the amount of paste food.

Word list： apply,　worrying,　proceeding,　increase,　keep,　looked

Anatomy and Physiology   **The Skin**

Medical Terminology

acidity	酸性	lactate	乳酸
adipose cell (fat tissue)		mineral	ミネラル
	脂肪細胞、脂肪組織	nerve ending	神経終末
ammonia	アンモニア	nerve fiber	神経線維
angina pectoris	狭心症	nipple	乳頭
apocrine gland	アポクリン腺	odor	におい
armpit	腋窩	patch	貼付剤、貼り薬
asthma	喘息	physiological	生理学的な
bacterial	細菌の	sebaceous gland	皮脂腺
breast	乳房	sebum	皮脂
collagen	コラーゲン	sensation	感覚
dermis	真皮	stratified squamous epithelium	
eccrine gland	エクリン腺		重層扁平上皮
elastic fiber	弾性繊維	subcutaneous tissue (hypodermis)	
epidermis	表皮		皮下組織
evaporation	蒸発	sweat gland	汗腺
external auditory canal		transdermal	経皮的な
	外耳道	urea	尿素

11

Reading Comprehension

Based on the text below, please answer the following questions.

1. How many layers does the heaviest body organ have?

2. What is the tissue of the outermost layer of skin?

3. What are the main components of the innermost layer of skin?

4. Where do you find the sweat glands?

5. What causes body odor?

6. What is the ideal acidity level for skin condition?

7. How is one's temperature controlled in the skin?

8. For what diseases can transdermal adhesive patches be used to treat?

The skin is the largest body organ in terms of surface area and weight. It is composed of three layers. The outermost layer is called the epidermis, and it covers almost the entire body surface. The tissues of the epidermis are stratified squamous epithelium which securely cover the body. The dermis is the middle layer of the skin and some of its structural components include collagen and elastic fibers. Blood capillaries, nerve fibers, and sebaceous glands are present in the dermis. The innermost layer of the skin is subcutaneous tissue (hypodermis) and its main components are adipose cells (fat tissue). Subcutaneous tissue contains larger blood vessels and nerves compared to those found in the dermis, where they become thinner.

Sweat glands are located in the dermis or the subcutaneous tissue and have openings on the epidermis that excrete sweat. There are two kinds of sweat glands: eccrine glands and apocrine glands. The eccrine glands are distributed in the skin throughout the body. The apocrine glands develop in the armpit, the area around the nipples of the breast and the external auditory canal during adolescence. The sweat from the apocrine glands is rich in fats and proteins and is the source of body odor.

The skin has five main physiological functions.

1. Protection of the internal body: The skin forms a barrier against bacterial infection and prevents dryness, keeping a condition of weak acidity (pH 5.5 - 7.0).

2. Regulation of temperature: The skin helps regulate several aspects of physiology including body temperature. Body temperature is controlled by the amount of blood flowing in the skin and through evaporation of sweat.

3. Excretion of wastes: The main component of sweat is water and it is secreted from sweat glands. Sweat helps eliminate excessive minerals, ammonia, urea, lactate, and sebum.

4. Receptor of sensations: Nerve endings at the dermis and subcutaneous tissues respond to temperature, pressure, and pain.

5. Absorption of particles: Fine particles such as smoke and moisture are absorbed through the skin. Currently, numerous transdermal patches are available such as ones used for treatment of asthma and angina pectoris. They are adhesive patches that are placed on the skin to deliver medication into the bloodstream through the skin.

Figure 1. 皮膚に関して、空所に適切な英語、あるいは<u>日本語</u>を記入しなさい。

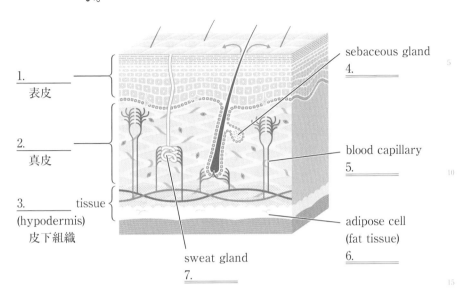

1. _____
   表皮

2. _____
   真皮

3. _____ tissue
   (hypodermis)
   皮下組織

sebaceous gland
4. _____

blood capillary
5. _____

adipose cell
(fat tissue)
6. _____

sweat gland
7. _____

Exercise 1. 本文の要約となるように下の語群より適語を選び、空所を補充しなさい。

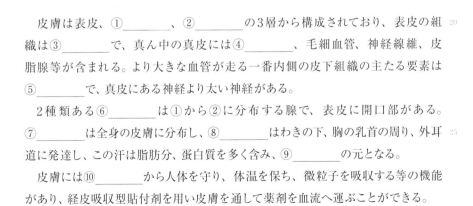

　皮膚は表皮、①_____、②_____の3層から構成されており、表皮の組織は③_____で、真ん中の真皮には④_____、毛細血管、神経線維、皮脂腺等が含まれる。より大きな血管が走る一番内側の皮下組織の主たる要素は⑤_____で、真皮にある神経より太い神経がある。

　2種類ある⑥_____は①から②に分布する腺で、表皮に開口部がある。⑦_____は全身の皮膚に分布し、⑧_____はわきの下、胸の乳首の周り、外耳道に発達し、この汗は脂肪分、蛋白質を多く含み、⑨_____の元となる。

　皮膚には⑩_____から人体を守り、体温を保ち、微粒子を吸収する等の機能があり、経皮吸収型貼付剤を用い皮膚を通して薬剤を血流へ運ぶことができる。

語群：皮下組織、体臭、細菌感染、コラーゲン線維、脂肪組織、真皮、
　　　重層扁平上皮、汗腺、エクリン汗腺、アポクリン汗腺

Exercise 2. 　皮膚の5つの機能について下記を補充しなさい。

		English	日本語
5	1	Protection of the ①＿＿＿＿ body, forming a barrier against bacterial ②＿＿＿＿ and keeping a skin condition of weak acidity	細菌感染に対する⑬＿＿＿＿機能として人体内部の保護、および皮膚の⑭＿＿＿＿の状態の保持
10	2	Regulation of ③＿＿＿＿, controlled by the amount of blood flowing in the skin and through evaporation of ④＿＿＿＿	皮膚を流れる⑮＿＿＿＿、および発汗を通じた、体温の調整
15	3	Excretion of ⑤＿＿＿＿, eliminating ⑥＿＿＿＿ minerals, ammonia, urea, ⑦＿＿＿＿, and sebum	過度のミネラル分、アンモニア、⑯＿＿＿＿、乳酸、⑰＿＿＿＿などの老廃物の⑱＿＿＿＿
	4	Receptor of ⑧＿＿＿＿, including temperature, pressure and ⑨＿＿＿＿	⑲＿＿＿＿、⑳＿＿＿＿、痛みなどの感覚の受容体
20	5	Absorption of ⑩＿＿＿＿, such as smoke, ⑪＿＿＿＿, and some kinds of ⑫＿＿＿＿	㉑＿＿＿＿や水蒸気、さらにはある種の薬剤といった微粒子の㉒＿＿＿＿

Unit 12

The Endocrine System
【内分泌系】

本課の ねらい	Dialog	糖尿病、血液透析や臨床工学技士に関する表現が使える。
	Anatomy and Physiology	内分泌の各分泌腺と働きに関する英語表現を理解する。

Dialog　Complications of Diabetes and Clinical Engineers

Medical Terminology

clinical engineer	臨床工学技士	pulse	脈拍
dialysis	透析		生命徴候（通常、血圧、脈拍、呼吸、体温をいう）
dialysis shunt	シャント	vital sign	
potassium	カリウム		

Reading Comprehension

Based on the dialog below, please answer the following questions.

1. How did the website help Ken when he left his lunchbox at home?
2. How much salt does curry contain according to the website?
3. How much salt did Ken take when he had a cutlet with a tablespoonful of ketchup?
4. What did the doctor advise Ken about his diet?
5. How does Ken clear up the waste in his blood?
6. What improvements did Ken's dialysis bring to Emma's cooking?
7. Where do clinical engineers work in the hospital?
8. Why did the clinical engineer say to Ken, "you are a model patient"?

Ken (58 years old) who has recently started dialysis, is talking about his diet with Emma (54 years old). 最近、透析を始めたKen (58歳) は食事についてEmma (54歳) と話し合っている。

₅
Emma： You left the lunchbox, and I was worrying about what you had for lunch.

Ken： Oh, I went to a restaurant for lunch today. The website you showed me was very useful in helping me choose dishes from the menu.

Emma： It is convenient to check what kind of nutrients a certain dish contains in a meal, isn't it?

Ken： It really is! I wanted to have curry and checked its nutrients at the website.

Emma： Curry contains more salt than you expected, doesn't it?

Ken： How do you know? According to the site, curry contains 3.99 grams of salt.

Emma： It is almost two thirds of your preferred salt amount per day.

Ken： So, the second choice was a pork cutlet, which has only 0.78 grams of salt.

Emma： That is only when you do not put sauce on it.

Ken： I ate a cutlet with only about a spoonful of ketchup.

Emma： Good for you! The salt in a tablespoonful of ketchup is 0.5 grams.

Ken： I have gotten used to less salty food lately. And I ate salad with vinegar.

Emma： How about potassium and phosphorus?

Ken： Potassium in a cutlet and salad is about two thirds of that in curry and phosphorus is much less in a cutlet than in curry.

Emma： Very good. And according to the doctor's advice, you can now have a diet containing more protein which was once restricted. With the help of dialysis, you can purify the waste products in the blood now.

Ken：　That is right. I can enjoy having food with protein and the waste is cleared by dialysis now. I am glad that I can eat more meat!

Emma：　You have been doing very well on your diet, exercise and medication.

Ken：　I was able to manage the situation only because you supported me in every aspect. 5

Emma：　But I wish we had noticed your diabetes earlier, then you could have avoided dialysis. I regret that.

Ken：　Let us be positive. I can keep myself in good condition with dialysis.

Emma：　That is true. Thanks to your well-regulated life, I can also keep a healthier lifestyle. I cook with less salt and many vegetables which is 10 good for both of us.

Ken：　I appreciate your great cooking. I would love to eat your curry.

Emma：　OK. I will cook special curry for your lunchbox tomorrow.

A clinical engineer (CE) is talking with Ken while preparing Ken's dialysis. 臨 15 床工学技士 (CE) がKenの透析の準備をしながらKenと話している。

CE：　Good evening. I'm Fukube, a clinical engineer. May I ask your name?

Ken：　I am Ken Yamahara. Nice to meet you. A clinical engineer?

CE：　Yes, as well as a nurse, we have the qualification to take care of dialy- 20 sis.

Ken：　I am afraid this is the first time I have seen a clinical engineer.

CE：　That's not surprising. Most of our work is done in the operating room in hospitals.

Ken：　There was a popular medical drama on TV in which a clinical engineer 25 was managing medical equipment during operations.

CE：　Thanks to the drama, our job in the operating room came to be known widely. Do you remember that we also work in the ICU and patients' rooms regulating the bedside equipment?

Ken：　I remember some staff member who was not a nurse visited me and 30 checked some equipment while I was in the hospital to put the shunt.

12

CE： Yes, that staff member must have been a CE. OK, now let me ask your body weight.

Ken： Here is the record of my body weight today.

CE： Thank you. Your weight is just the same as last time. Let me also take your pulse, blood pressure and temperature.

Ken： Yes, please take my vital signs.

CE： Your pulse is 62, blood pressure 132 over 86, and temperature 36.7 degrees Celsius. Have you had any health problem since the last dialysis?

Ken： Nothing in particular. I walk about an hour every day, keep a healthy diet and take medicine for diabetes and diabetic nephropathy.

CE： You are a model patient. Let me see around the dialysis shunt.

Ken： It is on my left arm. I have no problem on my skin, I think.

CE： I see. I will take your pulse … Good. I do not notice anyting abnormal. Let me put this rubber band around your arm. I will rub it with alcohol and insert the needle.

Ken： OK.

Exercise 1.　**Indicate True or False based on the dialog.**

会話文の内容に合っていればT、合っていなければFと記入しなさい。

( ) 1.　Curry contains less phosphorus compared to a cutlet.

( ) 2.　Ken is happy that he can eat more meat.

( ) 3.　Ken will probably have Emma's curry for lunch on the following day.

( ) 4.　Ken's pulse was not normal.

Exercise 2.　**The following is a report about Ken written by the CE. Fill in the blanks with words from the list.**

臨床工学技士が書いたKenについての報告です。空所を語群の語で埋めなさい。

Ken seems to have (1.　) in regular exercise, maintained healthy (2.　) and taken proper medication. He has no problem with his body (3.　), skin around the (4.　), and vital signs. He didn't know that a CE can handle (5.　), however, he understood our jobs and was cooperative.

Word list：shunt, engaged, dialysis, diet, weight

Anatomy and Physiology　**The Endocrine System**

Medical Terminology

acromegaly	先端巨大症	**ovary**	卵巣
adrenal	副腎(の)	**overproduction**	過剰産生
adrenal medulla	副腎髄質	**parathyroid**	上皮小体(の)
adrenalin	アドレナリン	**pineal**	松果体(の)
Basedow's disease	バセドウ病	**pituitary**	下垂体(の)
blood sugar	血糖	**reproduction**	生殖
concentration	濃度	**secrete**	分泌する
hormone	ホルモン	**testis**	精巣 (複数形はtestes)
human growth hormone	ヒト成長ホルモン	**TH (thyroid hormone)**	甲状腺ホルモン
hypersecretion	分泌過多	**thyroid**	甲状腺(の)
hypothalamus	視床下部	**TRH (thyrotropin-releasing hormone)**	甲状腺刺激ホルモン放出ホルモン
insulin	インスリン		
islets of Langerhans	ランゲルハンス島	**TSH (thyroid-stimulating hormone)**	甲状腺刺激ホルモン
malfunction	機能不全	**underproduction**	過少産生
noradrenalin	ノルアドレナリン		

12

Reading Comprehension

Based on the text below, please answer the following questions.

1. From where to where are hormones secreted?
2. What physical functions can be regulated by a small amount of hormones?
3. In what condition does diabetes occur?
4. What parts of body organs are responsible for diabetes?
5. What does hypersecretion of the thyroid hormone cause?
6. Where is growth hormone secreted from?
7. What is the relationship between a hormone's secretion and blood?
8. What does TSH (thyroid-stimulating hormone) lead to?

    The endocrine system is the collection of endocrine glands from which hormones, complex chemical substances, are secreted into the bloodstream. Although the amount of hormones secreted is very little, they can affect specific receptors significantly and regulate physical functions such as metabolism, growth and reproduction. Typical endocrine glands include the pituitary, pineal, thyroid, parathyroid and adrenal glands, as well as hypothalamus, islets of Langerhans, ovaries and testes. Even with a small change in the level of hormone secretion, either overproduction or underproduction, some serious diseases are triggered.

    One of the diseases related to the endocrine system is diabetes. Diabetes is a condition when the body cannot produce insulin or cannot use it efficiently. More specifically, it is the islets of Langerhans within the pancreases that are responsible for this condition. Basedow's disease and acromegaly are other examples that are caused by a malfunction of the endocrine system. Hypersecretion of the thyroid hormone from the thyroid gland causes Basedow's disease, while hypersecretion of human growth hormone from the anterior part of the pituitary gland results in acromegaly.

    The following is how hormonal secretion is regulated:

1. Changes in the concentration of chemical substances in the blood: For example, insulin is secreted from the pancreas when the concentration of blood sugar rises.

2. Control of the autonomic nerves: Adrenalin or noradrenalin is secreted from the adrenal medulla when the sympathetic nerve is activated.

3. Stimulation of other hormones: For instance, TRH (thyrotropin-releasing hormone), which is secreted from the hypothalamus, stimulates the anterior part of the pituitary gland where TSH (thyroid-stimulating hormone) is secreted. Then TH (thyroid hormone) is secreted from the thyroid gland.

4. Control of the feedback mechanism: This mechanism works like a loop in which a product (a certain type of hormone) feeds back to control its own production.

Figure 1.　内分泌に関して、空所1〜9に適する英語を答えなさい。

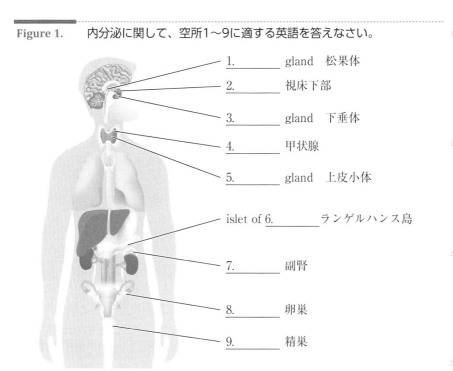

1.＿＿＿＿＿ gland　松果体

2.＿＿＿＿＿　視床下部

3.＿＿＿＿＿ gland　下垂体

4.＿＿＿＿＿　甲状腺

5.＿＿＿＿＿ gland　上皮小体

islet of 6.＿＿＿＿＿ランゲルハンス島

7.＿＿＿＿＿　副腎

8.＿＿＿＿＿　卵巣

9.＿＿＿＿＿　精巣

12

Exercise 1.　本文の要約となるように下の語群より適語を選び、空所を補充しなさい。

　内分泌系は①＿＿＿＿の集まりで、内分泌腺からホルモンは血流に分泌される。微量なホルモン分泌が特定の受容体に顕著に影響を与え、代謝、②＿＿＿＿、③＿＿＿＿といった身体機能を整える。典型的な内分泌腺には、④＿＿＿＿、松果体、⑤＿＿＿＿、上皮小体、⑥＿＿＿＿があり、⑦＿＿＿＿、⑧＿＿＿＿、卵巣、⑨＿＿＿＿といった器官の一部にもある。ホルモン分泌は様々な機構で調整され、過剰産生や不足といったわずかなホルモン分泌量の変化が、深刻な病気を引き起こすことがある。例として、膵臓の⑧から分泌されるインスリン不足が⑩＿＿＿＿を引き起こし、甲状腺ホルモンの分泌過多が⑪＿＿＿＿を、また、成長ホルモンの分泌過多が⑫＿＿＿＿を引き起こす。

語群：甲状腺、下垂体、視床下部、副腎、精巣、ランゲルハンス島、生殖、成長、バセドウ病、先端巨大症、糖尿病、内分泌腺

Exercise 2.　ホルモン分泌の4つの主な調整機能について下記の空欄を補充し、英語と日本語でまとめなさい。

	Hormonal secretion	Hormone examples	ホルモン分泌	ホルモン例
1	①＿＿＿＿in the concentration of chemical substances in ②＿＿＿＿	③＿＿＿＿	血中の化学物質の ⑪＿＿＿の変化	インスリン
2	Control of the ④＿＿＿＿nerves	adrenalin, ⑤＿＿＿＿	自律⑫＿＿＿による調整	⑬＿＿＿＿、ノルアドレナリン

3	⑥_____ of other hormones	TRH (thyrotropin-releasing hormone) →TSH (⑦_____ _____ _____) →⑧_____ hormone	他の⑭_____ による刺激	⑮_____ _____ →甲状腺刺激ホルモン →甲状腺ホルモン
4	⑨_____ of the ⑩_____ mechanism		フィードバック ⑯_____ による調節	

Unit

13

The Reproductive System
【生殖器系】

本課の ねらい	Dialog	前立腺がん、前立腺肥大症や看護師に関する表現が使える。
	Anatomy and Physiology	生殖器の構造と受精卵の発育に関する英語表現を理解する。

Dialog   Prostatic Hypertrophy and Nurses

Medical Terminology

antigen	抗原	rapport	ラポール、信頼関係
biopsy	生体組織検査、生検	tumor marker	腫瘍マーカー
digital rectal exam	直腸診	ultrasound	超音波(検査)
prostate cancer	前立腺がん	urinate	排尿する
prostatic hypertrophy	前立腺肥大症	urological	泌尿器科の
PSA (prostate specific antigen)			
	前立腺特異抗原		

Reading Comprehension

Based on the dialog below, please answer the following questions.

1. Why did Kenzo go to see a urologist?
2. How often does Kenzo urinate during the day?
3. What does Kenzo feel about his urination strength?
4. After talking to his wife, why did Kenzo feel scared about his urination?
5. How is a digital rectal exam performed?
6. What sample does Kenzo need to submit to check for his PSA level?
7. How is a biopsy conducted?
8. How can we communicate our feelings in addition to language use?

13

Susie (77 years old) is worried about Kenzo's (80 years old) frequent urination. Kenzo sees a urologist following her advice. Susie (77歳) はKenzo (80歳) の頻尿を心配し、その勧めで、Kenzoは泌尿器科を受診している。

Doctor： Hello, Mr. Yamahara. What seems to be the problem?

Kenzo： Nice to see you, Doctor. The problem is that I need to go to the restroom very often.

Doctor： How frequently do you urinate each day?

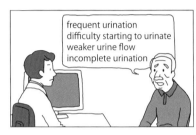

Kenzo： I go every hour and a half during the day and I wake up twice during the night to urinate, so about 12 or 13 times a day, I guess.

Doctor： Do you have difficulty starting to urinate?

Kenzo： Yes, a little. I need to strain my lower abdomen.

Doctor： Do you think it is difficult to maintain a steady stream of urine?

Kenzo： I'm not sure but my urination strength seems to have become weaker.

Doctor： Do you have any strange feeling after you finish urinating?

Kenzo： Well, I can't release my urine completely.

Doctor： Have you found any change in the color of your urine?

Kenzo： No. I don't think so. But my wife scared me when she said I might have prostate cancer! I hope it's something else!

Doctor： Well, the symptoms of prostate cancer and prostatic hypertrophy are similar. So, the next step is checking your urine flow. Then I'll check your prostate by inserting my finger into your rectum which is called a digital rectal exam.

Kenzo： Oh, no. It's horrifying but it's a necessary exam, isn't it?

Doctor： Yes. We also check the rectum using ultrasound and the PSA in your blood sample.

Kenzo： What is PSA?

Doctor：PSA is short for prostate specific antigen. It's a tumor marker.

Kenzo：If there is a PSA in my blood, does that mean I have prostate cancer?

Doctor：Not really. When the level is high, there's a possibility of prostate cancer. Then maybe next week, a biopsy will be carried out, in which your cells are examined by the microscope. Don't worry!

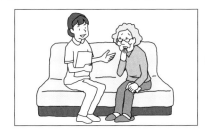

A registered nurse (RN) talks to Susie who is waiting for her husband in the urological waiting room. A nursing student (NS) is listening to their conversation.泌尿器科の待合室で待つSusieに、看護師 (RN) が声を掛ける。看護学生 (NS) がその会話を聞いている。

RN：   Are you OK?

Susie： I'm anxious about my husband's condition.

RN：   He's consulting with the doctor now, isn't he?

Susie： Yes. What shall I do if he has cancer?

RN：   Are you worried that his problem might be caused by cancer?

Susie： Yes. I cannot do anything without Kenzo, so if he has anything serious, I would cause too much trouble for the doctors and nurses.

RN：   I understand, but we will do what we can.

Susie： I also want to do something to help him, but I don't know what to do.

RN：   I know how you feel.

Susie： We have always been together and overcome everything together.

RN：   Yes, together. You can support him when he is ill.

Susie： Oh, I'm sure we can do anything together. Thank you, nurse.

The RN and an NS walked into the nursing station.

NS：   You never denied what she said even when cancer was something that she was thinking about.

RN： Sometimes it's necessary not to deny patients' uncertain utterances. The important thing is listening to her respectfully and letting her find the answers by herself.

NS： I understand. Your facial expressions were sympathetic and your voice sounded very sincere.

RN： We can convey our feelings with nonverbal communication, too. You learned a lot from our short conversation.

NS： Yes. I think it's important for co-medical staff to be sympathetic and sincere to build rapport with patients or family.

Exercise 1.　Indicate True or False and explain the reason.
会話文の内容に合っていればT、合っていなければFと記入しなさい。

( ) 1.　Kenzo feels that his urine stops before it is completely discharged.

( ) 2.　Kenzo understands a digital rectal exam is necessary to check his prostate.

( ) 3.　If a PSA is high, it means the person has prostate cancer.

( ) 4.　The registered nurse tells a nursing student that listening to patient's family respectfully and giving answers are always important.

Exercise 2.　The following is the NS's memo about the communication between Susie and a nurse. Fill in the blanks with words from the list.
以下は看護学生が患者の家族 (Susie) と看護師の会話から学んだことを書いたメモです。空所を語群の語で埋めなさい。

A patient's wife could find her answer by herself through verbal and nonverbal (1.   ) with a (2.   ). The co-medical staff's respectful (3.   ) and (4.   ) attitude is important to build (5.   ) between patients/family and co-medical staff.

Word list： nurse, communication, listening, rapport, sympathetic

Anatomy and Physiology The Reproductive System

Medical Terminology

accessory sex gland	付属生殖腺	ovulation	排卵
cell division	細胞分裂	ovum	卵子
embryo	胎芽	penis	陰茎
endometrium	子宮内膜	pregnancy	妊娠
estrogen	エストロゲン	progesterone	プロゲステロン
fallopian tube	卵管	prostate gland	前立腺
fertilization	受精	semen	精液
fertilize	受精させる	seminal vesicle	精嚢
fetus	胎児	sperm	精子
fimbria	卵管采	urinary bladder	膀胱、(単にbladderでも膀胱の意味で用いられる)
implant	着床する	uterus	子宮
mammary gland	乳腺	vagina	膣
menstrual cycle	月経周期	vulva	外陰部
menstruation	月経		

Reading Comprehension

Based on the text below, please answer the following questions.

1. What are organs of the female reproductive system? Name all of them in the strictest sense.
2. How long does an ovum usually stay in the uterine tube?
3. What could happen when an ovum meets a sperm cell in the fallopian tube?
4. How long does a fertilized ovum repeat cell division before it is implanted in the endometrium?
5. What is the usual menstrual cycle like for an adult woman?
6. At what age do females begin the secretion of estrogen and progesterone?
7. What do men's accessory sex glands do in the male reproductive system?
8. What is the main function of the male reproductive organs?

13

The female reproductive system is composed of internal organs including ovaries, fallopian tubes, uterus and vagina, and external organs such as the vulva. The uterus lies between the urinary bladder and the rectum and is connected to the outside of the body through the vagina. The breast is not a reproductive organ in the strictest sense, however, it can be defined as part of the female reproductive system because the mammary glands of a breast play an important role in the menstrual cycle, pregnancy and childbirth.

During the menstrual cycle, the ovum (egg) made in the ovary enters the fimbria of the fallopian tube at the time of ovulation and stays in the fallopian tube for two or three days. If it meets a sperm cell and is fertilized there, becoming a fertilized ovum, it starts a process of cell division. It repeats the division while moving to the uterus and it is implanted in the endometrium in 6 or 7 days after fertilization. When an ovum is not fertilized or a fertilized ovum fails to be implanted, endometrium is shed during menstruation. Normally in adult women, menstruation lasts for 3 to 5 days during the menstrual cycle of 24 to 36 days. In medical term, when the fertilized ovum is implanted, it is called the embryo and then the term becomes the fetus after passing the ninth week.

The ovaries secrete estrogen and progesterone. The estrogen secretion begins at about the age of eight or nine which creates women's characteristic body shape by storing fats under the skin, and developing female reproductive organs including mammary glands. Progesterone secretion begins at about 15 years of age when ovaries are mature, and it plays an important role in the menstrual cycle and pregnancy along with estrogen.

The male reproductive system consists of two testes, the duct system leading from them, the penis, and the accessory sex glands. Accessory sex glands, namely the seminal vesicles and prostate gland, produce secretions. Secretions from the seminal vesicles and prostate gland are mixed with the sperm from the testes to make semen. The main function of the male reproductive organs is the deposition of sperm within the female reproductive tract.

Figure 1.　　女性生殖器に関して、空所1〜5に適する英語を答えなさい。

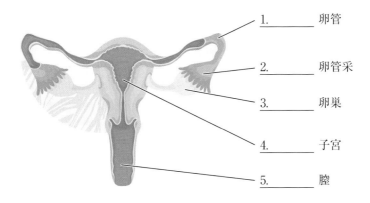

1. ＿＿＿＿＿　卵管

2. ＿＿＿＿＿　卵管采

3. ＿＿＿＿＿　卵巣

4. ＿＿＿＿＿　子宮

5. ＿＿＿＿＿　膣

Figure 2.　　男性生殖器に関して、空所1〜4に適する英語を答えなさい。

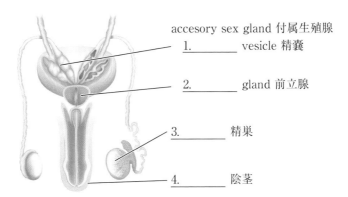

accesory sex gland 付属生殖腺

1. ＿＿＿＿＿　vesicle 精囊

2. ＿＿＿＿＿　gland 前立腺

3. ＿＿＿＿＿　精巣

4. ＿＿＿＿＿　陰茎

13

Exercise 1.　　本文の要約となるように下の語群より適語を選び、空所を補充しなさい。

　女性生殖器系には体内にある①＿＿＿＿＿、②＿＿＿＿＿、③＿＿＿＿＿、膣と身体の外部の④＿＿＿＿＿が含まれる（乳房を含むことがある）。①で作られた卵子は排卵後、⑤＿＿＿＿＿で受け取られ、②に2〜3日とどまる。この間に精子と出合い受精すると、受精卵は分裂を繰り返しながら③にたどり着き、受精後6〜7日で

⑥＿＿＿＿＿に着床し⑦＿＿＿＿＿となり、着床後、9週を過ぎると⑧＿＿＿＿＿と呼ばれるようになる。受精や着床が起こらなければ子宮内膜が剥がれ落ち⑨＿＿＿＿＿となり、通常このような月経周期は24〜36日である。卵巣では排卵の他、ホルモンが分泌される。⑩＿＿＿＿＿は8、9歳頃から分泌され、皮下脂肪を蓄えて女性らしい体を作り、さらに15歳頃からは⑪＿＿＿＿＿が分泌され月経および妊娠の成立と維持に重要な役割を果たす。

　　男性生殖器は2つの⑫＿＿＿＿＿、管、陰茎、付属生殖器である⑬＿＿＿＿＿と⑭＿＿＿＿＿から成る。⑫で作られた精子は付属生殖器で産生された分泌物と交じり合い精液となる。

語群：子宮、卵巣、卵管采、卵管、子宮内膜、月経、外陰部、胎芽、胎児、
　　　エストロゲン、プロゲステロン、前立腺、精嚢、精巣

Exercise 2.　　次の文章が本文の内容に合っているならTを、合っていなければFをそれぞれ記入しなさい。

( )1.　It takes 6 or 7 days for the fertilized ovum to be implanted.

( )2.　An ovum generated in the ovary moves to the fimbria of the fallopian tube.

( )3.　The ovum meets a sperm cell in the uterus.

( )4.　The fertilized ovum repeats the division.

( )5.　The menstrual cycle is from 3 to 5 days for a healthy adult woman.

( )6.　A womanly body develops by estrogen.

( )7.　Progesterone serves in the menstrual cycle and pregnancy.

( )8.　Semen is a compound made of sperm and secretions from the seminal vesicles and prostate gland.

Unit 14

The Immune System
【免疫系】

本課の ねらい	Dialog	じんましんや薬剤師に関する表現が使える。
	Anatomy and Physiology	免疫の種類としくみに関する英語表現を理解する。

Dialog   Hives and Pharmacists

Medical Terminology

acute	急性の	pharmacist	薬剤師
antihistamine	抗ヒスタミン薬	pimple	吹き出物、にきび
anti-itch	かゆみ止めの	pregnant	妊娠している
chronic	慢性の	rash	湿疹
histamine	ヒスタミン	side effect	副作用
hives	じんましん	welt	みみず腫れ

Reading Comprehension

Based on the dialog below, please answer the following questions.

1. What will scratches leave on Kay's skin?

2. Why hasn't Kay visited a dermatologist for her rashes?

3. How did Kay feel when she thought of her sleepless nights?

4. Where did Kay go at night instead of a clinic?

5. How did Kay explain her rashes well to a pharmacist at a drugstore?

6. How often does Kay's itchiness occur a day?

7. What medicine will the pharmacist give Kay?

8. What will Kay do if she has any side effects after taking the medicine?

14

Kay (29 years old) is talking about her hives with Ryuta (31 years old). Kay (29 歳) はじんましんについて Ryuta (31 歳) と話し合っている。

Ryuta：　You are scratching again. What's the matter?

Kay：　It's itchy all over my body. It may be hives. Would you look at my back?

Ryuta：　Let me see. Wow, there are rashes all over your back.

Kay：　I don't think I have eaten anything bad. I ate the same foods as you did.

Ryuta：　Stop scratching now. Scratches will leave red welts. Shall I put on some cream?

Kay：　I put on anti-itch cream as far as my hand could reach. The cold cream was comfortable, although it didn't seem to work on the rashes.

Ryuta：　OK. I'll put some cream on your back. Isn't it better to see a dermatologist?

Kay：　Well, they were so itchy the night before yesterday that I was thinking of going to the clinic the first thing in the morning.

Ryuta：　What did the dermatologist say?

Kay：　I didn't go because the rashes had disappeared completely when I woke up.

Ryuta：　But there are so many of them now.

Kay：　Yes. I thought they wouldn't come again but they reappeared in the evening. They come and go from time to time.

Ryuta：　It's Saturday and it doesn't seem serious enough to go to the emergency room.

Kay：　I know they are not fatal but I feel gloomy when I think of sleepless nights.

Ryuta：　Sleepless nights must be terrible. You should go to the clinic the day after tomorrow. I'll take a picture of your back with the rashes now. Then it will be easier to explain.

Kay：   That's a good idea! Take a picture of my back with my smartphone.

Ryuta： OK. Say cheese! Just joking. I took a good photo.

Kay：   Let me see...Wow, the massive rashes look like a map.

Ryuta： Well said! Just like a plateau. Do you think a drugstore is open now?

Kay：   I'm sure they close at 10 pm. They may have good medicine for my
          symptom.

Ryuta： I'll be taking care of children so go to see a pharmacist with the cell-
          phone.

Kay is talking with a pharmacist (PHAR) in a drugstore. Kayはドラッグストアで
薬剤師 (PHAR) と話している。

PHAR：   How can I help you?

Kay：   I had rashes all over my body.
          It may be hives but I can't think
          of anything that might have
          caused them.

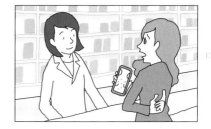

PHAR：   Can I have a look at the rashes?

Kay：   They have disappeared. They were everywhere and itchy just 10 min-
          utes ago.

PHAR：   What kind of rashes did you have?

Kay：   They are not small pimples and they spread like a map. My husband
          described them as plateaus. Oh, wait. There is a picture on my smart-
          phone.

PHAR：   That would be helpful. Let me see... They don't seem to be insect bites
          or atopic dermatitis.

Kay：   I agree with you. They were so itchy that I couldn't sleep well.

PHAR：   How long have you had the symptom?

Kay：   I have had the itchiness for a few days. It comes and goes a couple of
          times a day.

PHAR：   Your rashes are not chronic but acute... We can't diagnose, but they

14

seem to be caused by histamine released from some cells.

Kay： Why is histamine released?

PHAR： It may be induced by various conditions such as infection, medication, insect bites, food, psychological stress, or cold temperature.

Kay： I don't think I've experienced any of that...I'm not sure about stress, though.

PHAR： It is also said that the immune system or nervous system has something to do with the symptom. In many cases, it is hard to pinpoint the cause.

Kay： Is that so? Even if the cause is unclear, would you give me some medicine to stop the itchiness?

PHAR： Generally, antihistamines are the first choice for hives.

Kay： Then, I'll take the antihistamines to stop the irritating symptom.

PHAR： Are you pregnant?

Kay： No. But I am breast-feeding.

PHAR： That's very important information. Well then, this kind of antihistamines is safe for women who are breast-feeding. Have you had an allergic reaction after taking some medication?

Kay： No.

PHAR： If you experience any side effects indicated on the package, stop taking the medicine and consult a doctor, please.

Exercise 1.   Indicate True or False based on the dialog.

会話文の内容に合っていればT、合っていなければFと記入しなさい。

( ) 1.   Kay put anti-itch cream all over her back by herself.

( ) 2.   Kay thinks that she should go to the emergency room because of the rashes on her body.

( ) 3.   Kay cannot think of any cause for the rashes.

( ) 4.   There are various reasons why histamine is released.

Exercise 2. **The pharmacist (PHAR) is reviewing Kay's case. Fill in the blanks with words from the list.**

薬剤師がKayの事例を見直している。空所を語群の語で埋めなさい。

The cause of the client's (1.　) seemed like neither insect bites nor (2.　) dermatitis. Based on the shape and the timing of occurrence, they are probably caused by (3.　). She doesn't have a history of drug (4.　), but she is breast-feeding a baby. A good medicine was selected for her and advice about (5.　) was given.

Word list： side effects, histamine, rashes, atopic, allergy

Anatomy and Physiology　**The Immune System**

Medical Terminology

acquired immune system	獲得免疫系	immune response	免疫反応
adaptive immune system	適応免疫系	immune system	免疫系
adaptive immunity	適応免疫	inborn	生まれつきの、生来の
AIDS (acquired immunodeficiency syndrome)	エイズ、後天性免疫不全症候群	innate immune system	自然免疫系
allergic reaction	アレルギー反応	lymphocyte	リンパ球
antibody	抗体	macrophage	マクロファージ
APC (antigen-presenting cell)	抗原提示細胞	NK cell (natural killer cell)	ナチュラルキラー細胞、NK細胞
B cell	B細胞	pathogen	病原体、微生物
carrier	キャリア、病原体などの保有者	phagocytosis	食作用
cytotoxic T cell	細胞傷害性T細胞、キラーT細胞(killer T cell)ともいう	symptom	症状
foreign object	異物	T cell	T細胞
helper T cell	ヘルパーT細胞	transplant rejection	移植拒絶反応、移植片拒絶反応
HIV (human immunodeficiency virus)	ヒト免疫不全ウイルス	tumor	腫瘍
		virus	ウイルス

14

Reading Comprehension

Based on the text below, please answer the following questions.

1. At a micro level, what are the constituents of the immune system?
2. What does the immune system do at first when a body recieves a certain substance from the environment?
3. How does the immune system respond to harmful invaders?
4. What is antigen?
5. What causes allergic reactions?
6. What are two types of immune systems?
7. What substances become antigen-presenting cells (APCs)?
8. What are the two main types of T cells?

　　The immune system protects the body from harmful invaders in the environment, and it serves vital functions for the body. It consists of different organs, cells and proteins. We should know some kinds of lymphocytes called natural killer cells or NK cells, T cells and B cells and a kind of leukemia named macrophages among the constituents of the immune system. The immune system mainly works in two steps. The first step involves a recognition phase in which the immune system tries to recognize whether a certain substance is a part of one's own body or the foreign objects such as pathogens and cancer cells. The second step is called the immune response, where the system responds to foreign objects and destroys or removes the pathogens from the body.

　　A substance which causes an immune response is called an antigen. Various things, even fruit, can become antigens and may cause an immune response. For instance, infectious diseases are caused by bacteria or viruses, allergic reactions are caused by food, pollen, medicines and others, and transplant rejections are caused by foreign objects. There are two types in the immune system: innate immune system and adaptive (or acquired) immune system. Innate immunity, which is an inborn mechanism, works as the front line of defense within a few hours of infection of pathogens while adaptive immunity turns on slower, taking from 4 to 7 days.

　　In the innate immune system, natural killer cells (NK cells) work as defense, as dose macrophage, which engulfs and digests an antigen in a process called phagocytosis. Such cells as macrophages and B cells remember the pathogen after the first encounter and become antigen-presenting cells (APCs). APCs are the basis of another type of the immune system, the adaptive immune system. When APCs are presented to T cells, T cells are activated. The two main types of T cells are the helper T 5 cells and the cytotoxic T cells, also known as the killer T cells. As the names imply, the helper T cells "help" other cells in the immune system, whereas the cytotoxic T cells or the killer T cells "kill" infected cells and tumors. More specifically, as a commander, the helper T cells order the B cells to produce a special protein (antibodies) to catch antigens. The helper T cells also order the cytotoxic T cells to destroy the antigens in 10 the body. On the other hand, some of the antigens are caught by the antibodies.

One of the diseases which weakens or destroys the immune system is AIDS (acquired immunodeficiency syndrome). It does not mean, however that a person who is infected with human immunodeficiency virus (HIV) always develop AIDS. He or she can be an HIV carrier without having symptoms for 2-10 years. 15

Figure 1. 免疫に関して、空所1～4に適する英語を答えなさい。

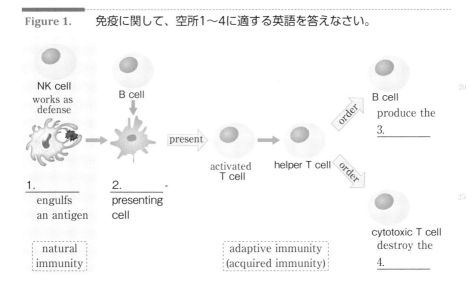

Exercise 1. 本文の要約となるように下の語群より適語を選び、空所を補充しなさい。

免疫とは体内に侵入した異物を見極め、それを攻撃し排除する機能のことである。さまざまな①＿＿＿＿＿を引き起こす物質を②＿＿＿＿＿と呼ぶ。例えば、③＿＿＿＿＿は細菌やウイルスによって引き起こされ、④＿＿＿＿＿は食物、花粉、薬剤等が抗原となる。免疫系には生まれながらにもっている⑤＿＿＿＿＿と、成長過程で得る⑥＿＿＿＿＿がある。前者はT細胞、B細胞等の⑦＿＿＿＿＿、白血球、白血球の一種の⑧＿＿＿＿＿が関わって感染を防ぐシステムで、後者は特定の病原菌との最初の接触により作り出された「記憶」によって、以降の接触の際には初回時よりも良い反応を導くものである。

T細胞には2種類あり、それぞれ、⑨＿＿＿＿＿と、細胞傷害性T細胞（⑩＿＿＿＿＿）と呼ばれ、免疫系においてヘルパーT細胞は他の細胞を「助ける」指令者であり、細胞傷害性T細胞は感染した細胞や腫瘍を破壊するという特徴がある。

> 語群：感染症、アレルギー反応、リンパ球、抗原、マクロファージ、獲得免疫系、
> 自然免疫系、免疫反応、ヘルパーT細胞、キラーT細胞

Exercise 2. 次の文章が本文の内容に合っているならTを、合っていなければFをそれぞれ記入しなさい。

( ) 1. The immune system in the body involves organs, cells and proteins.

( ) 2. The immune system has a step in which it destroys pathogens.

( ) 3. Fruit can be an antigen for causing an immune response.

( ) 4. Antigen-presenting cells are activated by T cells.

( ) 5. The helper T cells command the B cells to produce antibodies.

( ) 6. Those who carry HIV are always diagnosed with AIDS.

解答 編

Dialog
- Reading Comprehension
- Exercise の解答

Anatomy and Physiology
- Reading Comprehension
- Figure の解答
- Exercise の解答

Unit 1

Dialog

Reading Comprehension

1. Because she will have a medical checkup.
2. Because she was not able to make an appointment for the gastroscopy.
3. She will bring her samples for the fecal occult blood test, the application form, and the health insurance card.
4. She will take it in the hospital.
5. She has health insurance that is covered by Ken's company.
6. It is on the fifth floor.
7. It is at 9 o'clock.
8. Yes, she will. Because of a cancellation, she can have it.

Exercise 1 1. T   2. F   3. F   4. T   5. F
Exercise 2 1. an EGD   2. take   3. an appointment   4. an X-ray
5. a cancellation   6. change

Anatomy and Physiology

Reading Comprehension

1. It is the cell.
2. They are the skeletal, muscular, digestive, circulatory, respiratory, nervous, urinary, sensory, reproductive, endocrine, and the immune system.
3. They need to know the terms of position and direction.
4. It can be divided into the head and neck, the upper limbs, the back, the chest or thorax, the abdomen, the perineum, the pelvis, and the lower limbs.
5. It refers to the structures nearer to the front of the body.
6. It refers to the structures nearer to the feet.
7. The median plane.
8. It is anterior to the dorsal surface of the hand.

Figure 1 1. neck   2. 頭   3. upper   4. back   5. pelvis
6. limb   7. plane   8. thorax   9. 胸部   10. 腹部
11. 会陰   12. lateral   13. 内側

Figure 2 1. cranial   2. inferior   3. posterior   4. ventral   5. 背側
6. 前方   7. 上方   8. 尾側

Exercise 1 ①細胞 ②組織 ③器官 ④器官系 ⑤下肢 ⑥前方 ⑦後方
⑧頭側 ⑨尾側 ⑩正中面 ⑪外側 ⑫下方

Exercise 2

1. the skeletal system　　　　　骨格系
2. the digestive　　system　　消化器　系
3. the respiratory　system　　呼吸器　系
4. the nervous　　system　　神経　　系
5. the circulatory　system　　循環器　系
6. the urinary　　system　　泌尿器　系
7. the sensory　　system　　感覚器　系
8. the reproductive　system　　生殖器　系
9. the endocrine　system　　内分泌　系
10. the immune　　system　　免疫　　系
11. the muscular　system　　筋肉　　系

■ Unit 2

Dialog

Reading Comprehension

1. He/ She is a medical doctor who treats the bones and muscles.
2. The occupational therapist.
3. No, it won't.
4. By medication, exercise, and diet.
5. He suggested to Susie that she can walk to some places in her daily life.
6. He suggests to Susie to take a variety of food because calcium is included in various foods.

7. Vitamin D helps our body absorb the calcium and vitamin K develops bone formation.

8. Because vitamin D is produced by the sun's ultraviolet light.

Exercise 1 1. F 2. F 3. T 4. F 5. T

Exercise 2 1. pain 2. osteoporosis 3. medication 4. meals

5. anxiety 6. exercising 7. will

Anatomy and Physiology

Reading Comprehension

1. The cardiac, smooth, and skeletal muscles.

2. The skeletal and cardiac muscles.

3. It is attached to bone.

4. It can be seen in the walls of internal organs.

5. There are 206 bones in the adult human body.

6. They are a part of the skeletal system.

7. They produce blood cells.

8. They are classified as flat bones.

Figure 1 1. skeletal 2. cardiac 3. smooth 4. 横紋あり

5. striated 6. unstriated 7. voluntary 8. 不随意筋

9. involuntary 10. 蠕動

Exercise 1 ①横紋 ②収縮 ③平滑筋 ④蠕動 ⑤靭帯 ⑥骨髄 ⑦緻密骨

⑧海綿骨

Exercise 2 ①緻密骨の管 ②骨髄 ③上腕骨 ④ compact bone

⑤bone marrow ⑥femur ⑦radius ⑧ulna（⑥〜⑧順不同）

⑨薄い緻密骨 ⑩海綿骨の層 ⑪肩甲骨 ⑫compact bone

⑬spongy bone ⑭rib ⑮skull（⑭、⑮順不同）

Unit 3

Dialog

Reading Comprehension

1. Because she is constipated/She hasn't had a bowel movement for a few days.
2. He can use his hands to warm her stomach.
3. She will drink much water and take a laxative.
4. Vegetables contain a lot of fiber, which helps empty the bowels.
5. That afternoon.
6. It is prevention.
7. A dental technologist.
8. It is described as the brown line on the bottom of her teeth.

Exercise 1 1. F   2. T   3. F   4. T

Exercise 2 1. toothache   2. dentist   3. dental calculus   4. removing

Anatomy and Physiology

Reading Comprehension

1. It involves accessory organs.
2. It releases the nutrients of the food to be absorbed into the body.
3. The duodenum, jejunum, and ileum.
4. It is about 6 to 7 m long.
5. The tongue, salivary glands, pancreas, liver, and gallbladder.
6. It is the production of bile.
7. It is about 1.5 m long.
8. It is released into the duodenum.

Figure 1 1. oral cavity   2. pharynx   3. esophagus   4. stomach
5. pancreas   6. liver   7. gallbladder   8. small intestine
9. duodenum   10. jejunum   11. ileum   12. large intestine
13. cecum   14. ascending colon   15. transverse colon

16. descending colon   17. sigmoid colon   18. rectum

Exercise 1　①消化管　②膵臓　③食道　④酵素　⑤大腸　⑥肝臓　⑦胆嚢　⑧十二指腸

Exercise 2　1. F　2. F　3. F　4. T　5. T　6. F

■ Unit 4

▎Dialog

Reading Comprehension

1. She slept well for a few hours.
2. Because she has to breast-feed Naomi during the night.
3. She felt much better but she still felt dizzy and tired.
4. Because he wanted to see if she had anemia.
5. The results showed that her hemoglobin level was lower than the preferred level.
6. The doctor told her to consult with a registered dietitian first instead of taking medicine.
7. A good diet is helpful for some kinds of anemia.
8. At least 20 mg of iron per day are necessary.

Exercise 1　1. T　2. T　3. F　4. F

Exercise 2　1. hemoglobin　2. breast-feeding　3. iron　4. variety

▎Anatomy and Physiology

Reading Comprehension

1. It regulates body temperature.
2. Around pH 7.4 is regarded as being healthy.
3. There are erythrocytes or red blood cells, leukocytes or white blood cells, and platelets.
4. They serve an important part of the immune system as they help protect the body from infections.

5. It is made of water, salts, and protein.

6. The liquid part of blood.

7. They (these three elements) are included in plasma.

8. Some flow into lymphatic vessels.

Figure 1 1. plasma   2. clotting/coagulation   3. erythrocyte
4. leukocyte   5. platelet

Exercise 1 ①感染予防　②赤血球　③血小板　④血漿　⑤血清　⑥間質液
⑦リンパ管　⑧鎖骨下静脈

Exercise 2 1. T   2. F   3. F   4. F   5. T   6. F

Unit 5

Dialog

Reading Comprehension

1. Once a year. He has a chance to practice it in his company almost every year.

2. No, he hasn't. He has never performed it in real life.

3. We should pat his/her shoulders and ask him/her, "Are you OK?"

4. We should call an ambulance and start chest compression.

5. We should exhale air into the person's mouth while pinching his/her nose with our fingers.

6. It stands for automated external defibrillator.

7. They take X-rays and give radiation therapy.

8. It is to detect diseases of the lungs and the heart.

Exercise 1 1. F   2. F   3. F   4. T   5. F

Exercise 2 1. compression   2. ventilation   3. therapy   4. heart

Anatomy and Physiology

1. The heart.
2. The pulmonary and the systemic circulation.
3. The right ventricle.
4. It passes through the left ventricle.
5. The capillary.
6. They form the superior and inferior venae cavae.
7. Because the lymphatic vessels with lymph nodes lie just outside of the veins.
8. The former goes in one direction towards the heart, while the latter starts from the heart and returns to the heart.

Figure 1　1. pulmonary　　2. systemic　　3. capillary

Figure 2　1. superior　　2. right　　3. ventricle　　4. inferior　　5. aorta
　　　　　　6. artery　7. pulmonary　　8. atrium　　9. left

Exercise 1　①肺循環　②体循環　③右心室　④肺動脈　⑤左心房
　　　　　　⑥左心室　⑦大動脈　⑧細静脈　⑨リンパ節　⑩静脈

Exercise 2　1. F　　2. F　　3. F　　4. F　　5. F　　6. T

■ Unit 6

Dialog

1. It concentrates the oxygen out of the air.
2. Because with a nasal cannula, a person can breathe in oxygen as far as it reaches.
3. He puts a portable oxygen cylinder in a small cart.
4. He doesn't go out except to see a doctor.
5. His sister brings them every day.
6. Carrying a portable cylinder.

7. They talk, sing, play games and other such things.
8. Because he thought that people would be encouraged if he told them how he was doing with HOT.

Exercise 1　1. F　2. F　3. T　4. T
Exercise 2　1. visit　2. meals　3. interest　4. HOT　5. opportunity

Anatomy and Physiology

Reading Comprehension

1. It is composed of the lungs and the respiratory passages (respiratory tracts).
2. It is designed to exchange oxygen and carbon dioxide.
3. They make the glottis.
4. The bronchi.
5. The intimate relationship between pulmonary capillaries and alveolar air spaces.
6. They are the larynx and trachea.
7. They are mostly covered by a mucous film.
8. It serves as a chemical receptor for smell.

Figure 1　1. nasal　2. cavity　3. 咽頭　4. 喉頭　5. trachea
6. 右気管支　7. bronchus　8. artery　9. pulmonary
10. 細気管支　11. 毛細血管　12. 肺胞
Exercise 1　①気道　②気管支　③細気管支　④肺胞　⑤軟骨　⑥粘液
⑦組織　⑧化学受容体
Exercise 2　1. oxygen, carbon dioxide　2. pharynx, trachea, bronchioles, alveoli
3. capillaries, thin　4. mucous, respiratory, tissues
5. mucosa, smell　6. glottis, sounds

Unit 7

Dialog

Reading Comprehension

1. Because she felt annoyed by going to the restroom again.
2. We will feel less thirsty.
3. Our blood would thicken and could cause problems like a cerebral infarction.
4. He suggested drinking 100 mL of water 12 times, instead of drinking 200 mL of water 6 times.
5. She is sluggish in putting her shoes on or locking the door.
6. She made a rule to drink a half a glass of water every hour.
7. Because she went to the restroom every thirty minutes/She urinated so often.
8. Because seeing a small number of bacteria is so difficult that MTs increase the number to see them (bacteria) well.

Exercise 1 1. T   2. F   3. F   4. F
Exercise 2 1. advice   2. think   3. water   4. urination   5. doctor

Anatomy and Physiology

Reading Comprehension

1. It consists of two kidneys, two ureters, the bladder and the urethra.
2. They purify blood.
3. They are about 10 to 12 cm long, roughly the size of a large fist.
4. They are calyces and renal pelvises.
5. It surrounds a renal glomerulus.
6. It consists of the renal corpuscle and renal tubule.
7. It holds urine temporarily until it is excreted through the urethra.
8. A woman's urethra tends to be much shorter than a man's.

Figure 1 1. kidney   2. ureter   3. bladder   4. urethra   5. cortex

6. medulla　　7. 腎杯　　8. 腎盂

Figure 2　1. nephron　　2. 腎小体　　3. 尿細管　　4. ボウマン嚢　　5. 糸球体

Exercise 1　①腎臓　②尿管　③膀胱　④尿道 (①～④は順不同)　　⑤腎髄質
⑥腎皮質　⑦腎盂　⑧腎杯　⑨ネフロン　⑩糸球体　⑪ボウマン嚢
⑫腎小体

Exercise 2　1. blood, removed, bladder　　2. pH　　3. water, salt (順不同), filtrate
4. ureters, renal pelvis　　5. urethras

Unit 8

Dialog

Reading Comprehension

1. He was looking for his glasses.
2. Susie told him where they might be.
3. She often leaves her cellphone at home when she goes out.
4. She forgot their wedding anniversary.
5. It stands for mild cognitive impairment.
6. Because the online site about MCI says people should see a doctor early when they have unusual memory problems.
7. He did it perfectly.
8. He answered "a cat."

Exercise 1　1. T　　2. T　　3. F　　4. F

Exercise 2　1. subtraction　　2. numbers　　3. two　　4. recall
5. vegetables

Anatomy and Physiology

Reading Comprehension

1. It is called the nerve cell or neuron.
2. They are dendrites and an axon.
3. They are the central nervous system (the CNS) and the peripheral nervous

system (the PNS).

4. It contains a high density of cell bodies.

5. They are the cerebrum, cerebellum, and brain stem.

6. It serves as the center of most activities, sensations, and mental processes such as thought, intelligence, memory and language.

7. It controls the balance and movements of the body.

8. It connects the cerebrum and the spinal cord.

Figure 1 1. dendrite 2. cell body 3. axon

Figure 2 1. brain stem 2. diencephalon 3. mesencephalon 4. pons
5. medulla oblongata 6. cerebrum 7. 大脳皮質 8. 小脳
9. spinal cord

Exercise 1 ①中枢神経系 ②末梢神経系 ③ニューロン ④細胞体 ⑤軸索
⑥大脳 ⑦小脳 ⑧脳幹 ⑨大脳皮質 ⑩中脳 ⑪橋（脳橋）
⑫延髄（⑩〜⑫順不同）

Exercise 2 1. T 2. T 3. F 4. F 5. F 6. F 7. T

Unit 9

Dialog

Reading Comprehension

1. She hoped to burn body fat.

2. They saw leaves turning red and yellow, and found many acorns.

3. He bumped into a tree.

4. Because he had an unusual pain in his shoulder and was not able to move his arm.

5. Kay drove him there.

6. He has had his shoulder healing in a sling for three weeks.

7. Because he had not worked out much.

8. He should do it sixty times (in total).

Exercise 1　1. T　　2. F　　3. T　　4. T

Exercise 2　1. rehabilitation　　2. side　　3. shoulder　　4. hard　　5. continue
　　　　　　6. twice

Anatomy and Physiology

Reading Comprehension

1. It is made of all nerves that exist outside the brain and spinal cord.
2. They are the somatic nervous system and the autonomic nervous system.
3. They are sensory (afferent) and motor (efferent) nerves.
4. The sensory nerves bring information to the CNS, while motor nerves carry messages towards muscles, organs or other parts/The sensory nerves that receive information from external stimuli carry sensory information to the CNS, while motor nerves transmit impulses to contract muscles.
5. They are the cranial nerves and the spinal nerves.
6. There are 12 pairs.
7. They regulate the cardiac and smooth muscle activities, endocrine gland secretions, and the metabolism of certain cells.
8. They are called the sympathetic nervous system and the parasympathetic nervous system.

Figure 1　1. sensory　　2. motor

Figure 2　1. autonomic　　2. sympathetic　　3. parasympathetic　　4. rate
　　　　　　5. pressure

Exercise 1　①体性神経系　②自律神経系　③感覚神経　④運動神経　⑤脳神経
　　　　　　⑥脊髄神経　⑦心筋　⑧無意識　⑨交感神経　⑩副交感神経

Exercise 2　①末梢神経系　②体性神経系　③自律神経系　④感覚神経
　　　　　　⑤motor　⑥脳神経　⑦spinal　⑧31　⑨sympathetic
　　　　　　⑩副交感神経系

解答

Unit 10

Dialog

Reading comprehension

1. She has had them for two days.
2. She thinks that it is caused by a pollen allergy (such as cypress or other plants).
3. He told her to wash her hands completely with soap.
4. He told her that his pollen allergy had gotten better with acupuncture.
5. Neuralgia, rheumatoid arthritis and frozen shoulder.
6. She thinks that itchiness is the most problematic for her.
7. It depends on patients. Some patients feel the effect from the first time and others notice changes after several treatments.
8. Because the condition of the tongue gives the acupuncturist a lot of information about her.

Exercise 1 1. F 2. T 3. F 4. T

Exercise 2 1. itchy 2. diagnosed 3. conjunctivitis 4. acupuncture
5. effects

Anatomy and Physiology

Reading Comprehension

1. It converts the stimuli to impulses.
2. In the brain.
3. They construct the images that are promptly transmitted to the brain.
4. The retina.
5. It is located in the back of the brain in the area called the occipital lobes of the cerebrai contex.
6. Three.
7. The spiral organ of cochlea.
8. They are located at the sides of the brain in the area called the temporal

lobes of the cerebral cortex.

| Figure 1 | 1. cornea   2. anterior   3. pupil   4. lens   5. 硝子体 |

6. 網膜   7. 視神経

Figure 2	1. eye 2. optic nerve 3. 視交叉 4. 脳 5. 後頭葉
Figure 3	1. external 2. middle 3. internal 4. membrane 5. 蝸牛
Exercise 1	①インパルス ②瞳孔 ③網膜 ④視交叉 ⑤後頭葉 ⑥バランス

⑦鼓膜   ⑧アブミ骨   ⑨蝸牛   ⑩側頭葉

| Exercise 2 | 【光刺激】①前房   ②瞳孔   ③水晶体   ④網膜   ⑤視交叉 |

⑥cornea   ⑦pupil   ⑧vitreous body,   ⑨retina,   ⑩optic chiasm

【音波】①鼓膜   ②キヌタ骨   ③蝸牛   ④tympanic membrane

(eardrum)   ⑤the cochlea

Unit 11

Dialog

Reading Comprehension

1. They appeared last week.
2. She bought mittens.
3. He doesn't want Naomi to have atopic dermatitis.
4. She breast-feeds Naomi.
5. She has had baby food for two weeks.
6. Carrot paste was fed to her.
7. Kay should take her body to see a dermatologist even if when she takes care of her body's skin well and she has terrible rashes for a long time.
8. Because mittens prevent babies from controlling their temperature through their hands.

| Exercise 1 | 1. T   2. F   3. T   4. F |
| Exercise 2 | 1. worrying   2. looked   3. keep   4. apply   5. proceeding |

6. increase

解答

Anatomy and Physiology

Reading Comprehension

1. It has three layers.

5
2. It is the stratified squamous epithelium.

3. They are adipose cells (fat tissue).

4. We can find them in the dermis or the subcutaneous tissue (hypodermis).

5. The sweat from the apocrine glands.

6. Weak acidity between pH5.5-7.0 is ideal.

10
7. It is controlled by the amount of blood flowing (in the skin) and through evaporation of sweat.

8. Asthma and angina pectoris.

Figure 1　1. epidermis　　2. dermis　　3. subcutaneous　　4. 皮脂腺

15
　　　　　5. 毛細血管　　6. 脂肪細胞 (脂肪組織)　　7. 汗腺

Exercise 1　①真皮、②皮下組織 (①、②順不同)、③重層扁平上皮、④コラーゲン線維、⑤脂肪組織、⑥汗腺、⑦エクリン汗腺、⑧アポクリン汗腺、⑨体臭、⑩細菌感染

Exercise 2　English:①internal　②infection　③temperature　④sweat、

20
　　　　　⑤wastes　⑥excessive　⑦lactate　⑧sensations　⑨pain

　　　　　⑩particles　⑪moisture　⑫medicine

　　　　　日本語:⑬バリアー　⑭弱酸性　⑮血液　⑯尿素　⑰皮脂　⑱排出

　　　　　⑲体温　⑳圧力　㉑煙　㉒吸収

25
■ Unit 12

Dialog

Reading Comprehension

1. It helped him to choose dishes from the menu in the restaurant.

30
2. It contains 3.99 grams of salt.

3. He took 1.28 grams of salt. (0.78+0.5grams)

4. The doctor advised Ken to have a diet containing more protein than before.

5. With the help of dialysis he can purify the waste products in his blood.

6. She now cooks with less salt and many vegetables.

7. They work in the operating room, ICU, and patients' rooms.

8. Because Ken walks about an hour every day, keeps a healthy diet, and takes medicine for diabetes and diabetic nephropathy.

Exercise 1 1. F   2. T   3. T   4. F

Exercise 2 1. engaged   2. diet   3. weight   4. shunt   5. dialysis

Anatomy and Physiology

Reading Comprehension

1. They are secreted from endocrine glands to the blood stream.

2. Metabolism, growth and reproduction.

3. It occurs in a condition when the body cannot produce insulin or cannot use it efficiently.

4. The islets of Langerhans within the pancreas.

5. It causes Basedow's disease.

6. It is secreted from the anterior part of the pituitary gland.

7. A hormone's secretion changes in the concentration of chemical substances in the blood.

8. It leads to secretion of the thyroid hormone.

Figure 1 1. pineal   2. hypothalamus   3. pituitary   4. thyroid
5. parathyroid   6. Langerhans   7. adrenal   8. ovary
9. testis

Exercise 1 ①内分泌腺   ②成長   ③生殖（②、③順不同）   ④下垂体   ⑤甲状腺
⑥副腎（④-⑥順不同）   ⑦視床下部   ⑧ランゲルハンス島   ⑨精巣
（⑦、⑨順不同）   ⑩糖尿病   ⑪バセドウ病   ⑫先端巨大症

Exercise 2 ①Changes   ②blood   ③insulin   ④autonomic   ⑤noradrenalin
⑥Stimulation   ⑦thyroid-stimulating hormone   ⑧thyroid

解答

⑨Control　⑩feedback　⑪濃度　⑫神経　⑬アドレナリン
⑭ホルモン　⑮甲状腺刺激ホルモン放出ホルモン　⑯機構

Unit 13

Dialog

Reading Comprehension

1. Because he had to go to the restroom very often.
2. He urinates about 10 times during the day.
3. He feels that it has become weaker.
4. Because his wife Susie told him that he might have prostate cancer.
5. It is performed by inserting a doctor's finger into a patient's rectum.
6. He needs to submit his blood sample.
7. The cells are examined by the microscope.
8. We can convey them with nonverbal communication.

Exercise 1　1. T　　2. T　　3. F　　4. F
Exercise 2　1. communication　　2. nurse　　3. listening　　4. sympathetic
　　　　　　　5. rapport

Anatomy and Physiology

Reading Comprehension

1. The ovaries, fallopian tube, uterus, vagina and vulva.
2. It usually stays for two or three days.
3. It could be fertilized (becoming a fertilized ovum) and could start a process of cell division/Fertilization.
4. It repeats the division for six or seven days.
5. It is about a 24 to 36 day cycle.
6. Estrogen secretion begins at about the age of eight or nine, while progesterone secretion begins at about 15 years of age.
7. They produce secretions.

8. It is the deposition of sperm within the female reproductive tract.

| Figure 1 | 1. fallopian tube   2. fimbria   3. ovary   4. uterus   5. vagina |

| Figure 2 | 1. seminal   2. prostate   3. testis   4. penis |

| Exercise 1 | ①卵巣　②卵管　③子宮　④外陰部　⑤卵管采　⑥子宮内膜 |

⑦胎芽　⑧胎児　⑨月経　⑩エストロゲン　⑪プロゲステロン

⑫精巣　⑬精嚢　⑭前立腺（⑬、⑭順不同）

| Exercise 2 | 1. T   2. T   3. F   4. T   5. F   6. T   7. T   8. T |

Unit 14

Dialog

Reading Comprehension

1. Red welts will be left.

2. Because her rashes tend to disappear completely from time to time.

3. She felt gloomy when she thought of her sleepless nights.

4. She went to see a pharmacist at a drugstore.

5. She did it by showing the picture of her back on her smartphone.

6. It comes and goes a couple of times a day.

7. The pharmacist will give Kay an antihistamine.

8. She will stop taking the medicine and consult a doctor.

| Exercise 1 | 1. F   2. F   3. T   4. T |

| Exercise 2 | 1. rashes   2. atopic   3. histamine   4. allergy |

5. side effects

Anatomy and Physiology

Reading Comprehension

1. They are some types of lymphocytes, called natural killer cells or NK cells, T cells and B cells, as well as a kind of leukemia named macrophages.

2. It tries to recognize whether a certain substance is a part of one's own body

解答

or a foreign object.

3. It destroys or removes them.

4. It is a substance which causes an immune response.

5. Food, pollen, medicines and others.

6. They are innate immune system and adaptive (or acquired) immune system.

7. Macrophages and B cells.

8. The helper T cell and the cytotoxic T cell.

Figure 1　1. macrophage　　2. antigen　　3. antibodies　　4. antigens

Exercise 1　①免疫反応　②抗原　③感染症　④アレルギー反応　⑤自己免疫系
⑥獲得免疫系　⑦リンパ球　⑧マクロファージ　⑨ヘルパーT細胞
⑩キラーT細胞

Exercise 2　1. T　　2. T　　3. T　　4. F　　5. T　　6. F

一般に用いられる病名の医学英語

ア 行

悪液質	cachexia
悪性腫瘍	malignant tumor
悪性貧血	pernicious anemia
アデノイド	adenoid
アトピー性皮膚炎	atopic dermatitis
アフタ	aphtha
アフタ性口内炎	aphthous stomatitis
アルコール依存症	alcoholism
アルツハイマー病	alzheimer disease
アレルギー	allergy
アレルギー性鼻炎	allergic rhinitis
胃炎	gastritis
胃潰瘍	gastric ulcer
胃癌	gastric cancer
遺伝病	hereditary disease
咽頭炎	pharyngitis
インフルエンザ	influenza
ウイルス性肝炎	viral hepatitis
齲蝕	dental caries
うっ血	congestion;
うつ病	depression
うつ病メランコリー	melancholis
エプーリス	epulis
嚥下困難	dysphagy
嚥下性肺炎	aspiration pneumonia
炎症	inflammation
黄疸	jaundice

か 行

壊血病	scurvy
外傷	trauma
外傷性脱臼	traumatic dislocation

潰瘍	ulcer
顎関節症	temporomandibular arthrosis
過呼吸	tachypnea
風邪　感冒	common cold
家族性大腸腺腫症	familial adenomatous polyposis
化膿性骨髄炎	suppurative osteomyelitis
過敏症	hypersensitivity
花粉症	pollinosis , Hay fever
癌	cancer
肝炎	hepatitis
肝癌	liver cancer
肝硬変	liver cirrhosis
肝細胞癌	liver cell carcinoma, hepatocellular carcinoma
カンジダ症	candidiasis, candidiosis
癌腫	carcinoma
癌性腹膜炎	peritonitis carcinomatosa
関節炎	arthritis
関節リウマチ	rheumatoid arthritis
感染症	infectious disease
気管支炎	bronchitis
気管気管支炎	tracheobronchitis
気管支喘息	bronchial asthma
気管支肺炎	bronchial pneumonia
気胸	pneumothorax
寄生虫	parasite
逆流性食道炎	reflux esophagitis
急性の	acute
狭心症	angina pectoris

142

虚血性心疾患	ischemic heart disease		
近視	myopia		
筋ジストロフィー	muscular dystrophy		
クモ膜下出血	subarachnoidal hemorrhage		
くる病	rackets		
痙攣	convulsion		
結核	tuberculosis		
血管炎	vasculitis		
血栓症	thrombosis		
血尿	hematuria		
結膜炎	conjunctivitis		
血友病	hemophilia		
下痢	diarrhea		
健忘症	amnesia		
口蓋裂	cleft palate		
高血圧症	hypertension		
高血糖	hyperglycemia		
膠原病	collagen disease		
高脂血症	hyperlipemia		
甲状腺炎	thyroiditis		
甲状腺癌	thyroid cancer		
後天性免疫不全 deficiency 症候群	acquired immuno-syndrome（AIDS）		
喉頭癌	laryngeal cancer		
口内炎	stomatitis		
誤嚥性肺炎	aspiration pneumonia		
股関節　変形性 関節炎	osteoarthritis		
昏睡	coma		
黒子(ほくろ)	lentigo simplex		
骨腫瘍	bone tumor		
骨髄炎	osteomyelitis		
骨折	fracture		
骨粗鬆症	osteoporosis		
骨肉腫	osteoblastic sarcoma		

サ行

細菌性食虫毒	bacterial food poisoning
再生不良性貧血	aplastic anemia
坐骨神経痛	sciatica
痔	hemorrhoid
子宮外妊娠	ectopic pregnancy
子宮筋腫	myoma uteri
子宮頸癌	cervical cancer
子宮内膜癌	endometrium cancer
歯根嚢胞	radicular cyst
歯周炎	periodontitis
歯周病	periodontal disease
歯髄炎	pulpitis
失禁	incontinence
歯肉炎	gingivitis
自閉症	autism
出血	hemorrhage
腫瘍	tumor
静脈瘤	varix
褥瘡	decubitus ulcer
食道炎	esophagitis
食道癌	esophageal cancer
食道静脈瘤	esophageal varix
腎盂腎炎	pyelonephritis
腎炎	nephritis
心筋炎	myocarditis
心筋梗塞	myocardial infarction
神経痛	neuralgia
進行癌	advanced cancer
腎細胞癌	renal cell carcinoma
心臓弁膜症	valvular heart disease
心内膜炎	endocarditis
心肥大	cardiac hypertrophy
心不全	heart (cardiac) failure
蕁麻疹	urticaria

唇裂（兎唇）	cleft lip
膵炎	pancreatitis
膵臓癌	pancreatic cancer
水痘（みずぼうそう）	varicella , chicken pox
水疱	bulla
生活習慣病	lifestyle related disease
精神病	psychosis
性病	venereal　disease
舌癌	lingual cancer
喘息	asthma
先天奇形	congenital malformation
前立腺炎	prostatitis
前立腺癌	prostatic cancer
前立腺肥大	prostatic hyperplasia
早期癌	early cancer
創傷	wound
塞栓症	embolism
卒中	apoplexy

タ行

帯状疱疹	herpes zoster
大腸炎	colitis
大腸癌	cancer of the large intestine
ダウン症候群	down syndrome
唾液腺炎	sialadenitis （sialoadenitis）
唾石症	sialolithiasis
脱臼	luxation
脱水　脱水症状	dehydration
打撲	bruise
胆管炎	cholangitis
単純ヘルペス（口唇ヘルペス）	herpes simplex
胆石症	cholelithiasis

胆嚢癌	gallbladder cancer
中耳炎	otitis media
虫垂炎	appendicitis
腸閉塞	ileus
椎間板ヘルニア	intervertebral disc hernia
痛風	gout
低血圧（症）	hypotension
テタニー　硬直	tetany
鉄欠乏性貧血	iron deficiency anemia
転移	metastasis
統合失調症	schizophrenia
糖尿病	diabetes mellitus
動脈硬化症	atherosclerosis
動脈瘤	aneurysm
吐血	hematemesis

ナ行

肉腫	sarcoma
日本脳炎	Japanese B encephalitis
乳癌	breast cancer
乳腺炎	mastitis
乳腺症	mastopathy
尿道炎	urethritis
尿毒症	uremia
認知症	dementia
熱傷	burn
ネフローゼ症候群	nephrotic syndrome
捻挫	sprain, distortion
脳血栓症	cerebral thrombosis
脳梗塞	cerebral infarction
脳死	brain death
脳卒中	cerebral apoplexy
脳内出血	intracerebral hemorrhage

脳軟化症	encephalomalacia
囊胞腎	cystic disease of the kidney
脳膜炎	meningitis
膿瘍	abscess

ハ行

パーキンソン病	parkinson disease
肺炎	pneumonia
肺気腫	pulmonary emphysema
肺結核	pulmonary tuberculosis
敗血症	sepsis（septicemia）
梅毒	syphilis
白内障	cataract
麦粒腫（ものもらい）	hordeolum
破傷風	tetanus
バセドウ病（グレーブス病）	basedow disease（graves disease）
白血病	leukemia
鼻炎	rhinitis
皮膚炎	dermatitis
皮膚癌	skin cancer, cutaneous carcinoma
飛蚊症	myodesopsia
肥満症	obesity
日和見感染症	opportunistic infection
貧血	anemia
貧血	anemia
頻尿	pollakiuria
頻脈	tachycardia
風疹	rubella
腹水	ascites
腹膜炎	peritonitis
浮腫（水腫）	edema

不整脈	arrhythmia
変形性関節症	arthrosis deformans
扁桃炎	tonsillitis
便秘	constipation
膀胱炎	cystitis
膀胱癌	cancer of the urinary bladder
乏尿	oliguria
勃起不能症	impotence
発作　卒中	stroke
発疹	exanthem

マ行

麻疹（はしか）	rubeola, measles
慢性の	chronic
無意識状態	unconsciousness
無尿	anuria
メニエール病	ménière's disease
網膜剥離	retinal detachment

ヤ行

溶血性貧血	hemolytic anemia

ラ行

卵巣腫瘍	ovarian tumor
リウマチ熱	rheumatic fever
流行性耳下腺炎（おたふくかぜ）	mumps
良性腫瘍	benign tumor
緑内障	glaucoma
リンパ管炎	lymphangitis
リンパ節炎	lymphadenitis
淋病	gonorrhea
老化	senescence
老人性萎縮	senile atrophy
肋間神経痛	neuralgia

索 引
INDEX

150

〈編者略歴〉

小澤 淑子（こざわ　よしこ）

1977年　南山大学文学部英語学英文学科卒業
2003年　愛知県立看護専門学校卒業、看護師資格取得
2005年　岐阜大学大学院教育学研究科教科教育先行英語教育専修修了
2006年　Transworld Schools TESOL Advanced Course 修了
2015年　名古屋外国語大学大学院国際コミュニケーション研究科博士
　　　　後期課程（英語教育学分野）単位取得後退学
現　在　鈴鹿医療科学大学 看護学部看護学科 教授

医療従事者のためのベーシックイングリッシュ

2020年4月1日　　第1版第1刷発行

編　　者　小澤淑子
発行者　村上和夫
発行所　株式会社 オーム社
　　　　郵便番号　101-8460
　　　　東京都千代田区神田錦町3-1
　　　　電話　03(3233)0641（代表）
　　　　URL https://www.ohmsha.co.jp/

© 小澤淑子 2020

組版　トップスタジオ　　印刷・製本　壮光舎印刷
ISBN978-4-274-22489-8　Printed in Japan

本書の感想募集 https://www.ohmsha.co.jp/kansou/

本書をお読みになった感想を上記サイトまでお寄せください。
お寄せいただいた方には，抽選でプレゼントを差し上げます。

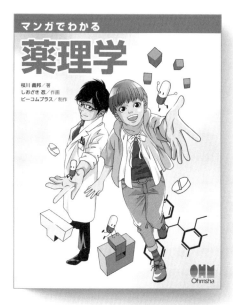